BACK TO BALANCE

Thank you for
getting Back to
Balance!

Best
Halee

BACK TO
BALANCE

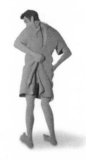

The Art, Science,
and Business of Medicine

DR. HALEE FISCHER-WRIGHT

DISRUPTION
BOOKS

AUSTIN   NEW YORK

Although some of the stories in this book are true, many of the names and identifying characteristics of the subjects have been changed to protect their privacy.

The views expressed by the author of this book are not intended as a substitute for medical advice, diagnosis, or treatment provided by the reader's personal physicians.

Published by Disruption Books
Austin, TX, and New York, NY
www.disruptionbooks.com

Distributed by Disruption Books

For ordering information or special discounts for bulk purchases, please contact Disruption Books at info@disruptionbooks.com.

Cover illustration by Gail Armstrong
Cover design by Lauren Harms
Text design by Kachergis Book Design

Print ISBN: 978-1-63331-014-8
eBook ISBN: 978-1-63331-015-5

10 9 8 7 6 5 4 3 2 1

Dedication

To the people of the medical practice: the patients, the providers, and especially the practice leaders. Thank you for inspiring me every single day.

To my parents who let me do whatever I wanted to do … 'cause I was gonna do it anyway. I love you both very much.

And to Michael — I love you more.

CONTENTS

CONTENTS

BACK TO BALANCE

CHAPTER I

Business in the Front, Party in the Back, and Common Sense Pushed Out the Door

What are the things we refuse
to talk about in health care and
why do they matter?

THERE'S BEEN A LOT OF TALK in recent years about something that has been the butt of more jokes than any other single aspect of America's health-care system.

It's been called "depersonalizing." It's been dismissed as "unflattering." It's been universally derided as "dreaded," "traumatizing," "misguided and malfunctioned," "horrible," "long hated and embarrassing," "demeaning," "humiliating," "uncomfortable," "least loved," and by one especially colorful southern woman, "ass-inine."

It is, as one doctor has described it, "health care's version of the prison jumpsuit." I'm talking of course about the original "business in the front and party in the back": the flimsy open-to-the-breeze, tie-in-the-back, itchy, pant-less, unisex, muted blue, standard-issue hospital gown.

You know it. It's the one said to come in three sizes: short, shorter, and "don't bend over." The one said to be like health insurance, because "you're never covered as much as you think you are."

But one thing that has rarely if ever been said about hospital gowns is that they are "the key to patient satisfaction" in health care—that is, until the e-newsletter *Healthcare Business & Tech-*

nology suggested as much in April 2015.[1] As a physician, I have to admit to being surprised by that idea, because I've always considered things like compassion and empathy and effective care that produces good results to be the key to patient satisfaction.

But it's not hard to understand the appeal. After all, we all have gown stories of our own.

While I was a medical student and working at a county hospital, I had what I thought was a stomach virus. After I'd been sick for a week, I suddenly went from "my stomach hurts" to "oh my God, I'm going to die." The doctor I was doing my rotation with actually drove me to the teaching hospital where many of my fellow medical students were working, which was a Level I Trauma Center. They took me into the ER, stripped me out of my clothes, and gave me a hospital gown.

Within a few minutes, seemingly everyone in my medical school class, along with other concerned doctors, came by to say hi and check in on what was diagnosed as an acute appendicitis. Problem was, my stomach was more focused on violently expelling everything that was in it. All I could think about was making my way to the bathroom on the other side of the room. As I got out of bed, I suddenly remembered that the gown was the only thing I was wearing. I couldn't figure out how to hold the top of me in place while keeping my gown closed in the back at the same time. I decided that I would be less embarrassed if they saw my backside than my boobs, crossed my arm against my chest, and ran to the bathroom.

A decade later, I had a similar incident. By then, I had become president of a large medical group associated with the hospital. I'd run a half marathon and gotten so dehydrated, I ultimately damaged my gallbladder, becoming seriously ill. Again, I went to the ER and was given a gown. I didn't care—I thought I was headed to the operating room. But then my surgery got delayed and I sat in pre-op for four hours.

Once again, my fellow doctors came in to check on me. One very loving friend leaned in a little too hard for a comically exaggerated hug and dislodged the delicate strings I had tied in the back. The gown came down and my friend was treated to the full Mardi Gras. I'm not sure what was more traumatic for him: the sight of me exposed or the horrible things I screamed at him.

For an item that has been the recipient of so much bad-mouthing, the humble hospital gown has shown remarkable staying power. It's been around longer than X-rays and antibiotics, Band-Aids and even private health insurance. And it's been remarkably resistant to change: We've basically gone from a gown with strings that only people who are double-jointed can tie, to a gown with snaps that come unsnapped at the slightest bit of pressure, to a gown with Velcro straps that never line up and rarely continue to stick after a few dozen washings.

The official reason given for the long prominence of these gowns is that they are easy to open and close, giving doctors and other health physicians the quick access they need to examine and treat patients. The unofficial reason for their longevity is that they are inexpensive and durable. Still, the fact remains that there are few times in life that we feel more vulnerable than when illness or injury force us into a hospital. It doesn't take a patient advocacy group to know that it's not optimal to then strip people nude and put them in what's been called "the most vulnerable garment ever invented."[2]

But a funny thing happened on the way to the twenty-first century: some gowns began to get a makeover. In 1999, New Jersey's Hackensack University Medical Center contracted with designer Nicole Miller to overhaul its gowns. In 2010, the Cleveland Clinic unveiled a new gown created by design legend Diane von Furstenberg. Hospitals from Michigan to Idaho to North Carolina to Missouri to Minnesota soon followed. All of a sudden, patients had the chance, as one writer put it, "to keep your pants, and your dignity, at the hospital."[3]

Why the sudden rush to create a more patient-friendly gown

after a century of disinterest? In a word, dollars. As *The Atlantic* explained in a 2015 story, "In recent years, hospitals are looking at everything they do and trying to evaluate whether or not it contributes to enhancing the patient experience.... The Centers for Medicare and Medicaid Services increasingly factors patients' satisfaction into its quality measures, which are linked to the size of Medicare payments hospitals get."[4]

In other words, the more that America's health-care institutions can do to make patients happier—from better gowns to more accessible parking to clearer corridor signs to better food to friendlier receptionists—the better their health scores will be and the better America's health-care system will be.

I'm pretty excited about this. I'm all for nicer gowns, closer parking spaces, and better food. It will definitely make the customer experience in our institutions of healing and medicine that much more civilized. It will make patients feel less like patients and more like people treated with greater dignity and respect.

It will also make it much friendlier and more comfortable for everyone when America's entire health-care system collapses in about a decade under the combined weight of all the things we keep refusing to talk about that are truly making patients, physicians, and medical practice administrators alike miserable today.

I give administrators props for at least trying to do *something* to make positive change in an industry where every attempt to make things better so often seems to make things worse. But I think we should stop settling for the kind of thinking that believes redesigning a hospital gown is "a big idea" for improving health care in America.

The problem isn't that hospital gowns are drafty—nor is it that health insurance companies are evil or physicians are money-hungry or hospitals are irresponsible or robots are taking over or patients are misguided or any of a hundred other reasons that have been used to sell books and win political campaigns over the past few decades. The problem, to paraphrase a point that Jon Stewart once made in a speech to his alma mater, is that while we were focused on yelling about all of those other things, we heard a pinging sound, and the thing just about died on us. We've asked a million questions, but we still haven't been asking the right questions. Why have we lost our focus on what matters most in health care?

We have lost our focus on strengthening the one thing that we know has always produced healthier patients, happier doctors, and better results: namely, strong relationships between patients and physicians, informed by smart science and enabled by good business, that create the trust necessary to ensure that patients do what they need to do to achieve the outcomes we all want from health care. Instead, we have reached a point of serious imbalance, and each new change that rolls through the industry just keeps layering more weight in all of the wrong places.

Health care works best when the art, science, and business of medicine are allowed to work in balance with one another—each doing its part *and no more* to help Americans get healthy and stay healthy. We've allowed that equilibrium to gradually, but increasingly, fall apart over the past thirty or forty years. We need to get it back.

This book is about how we bring the art, science, and business of medicine back to balance—and along the way, bring American health care back to excellence. For all of us.

The Heart of Medicine

When I close my eyes, there is another gown I see, and another patient, in another hospital, during a moment I will never forget.

I was wearing a short white lab coat, following along with my fellow medical students like ducklings behind our revered attending physician—easy to identify by his graying temples, his longer white coat, and his confident bearing at the head of the brood. He was leading us on rounds that morning, training us as we moved from patient to patient in a Denver hospital. We pushed into the next room, which reeked of that smell specific to hospitals—a combination of antiseptic and suffering. In the middle of this dingy room with shabby curtains was a normal-sized man sitting on a bed.

Against the backdrop of the room, he seemed scared and small. None of us said anything to him as we entered. The attending physician was the first to speak, "Here we have a forty-six-year-old man with possible multiple sclerosis. We're here today to do a spinal tap." No mention of the patient's name. No eye contact with the patient as the doctor pulled out a six-inch needle. None of us wanted to acknowledge how scared the man seemed. "We'll draw fluid from his spinal column and measure the amount of protein present in the fluid to determine how aggressively to treat the disease."

A senior resident, also responsible for our training, would attempt the procedure first—to show us how it was done. He moved to the bed and positioned the patient to sit on the edge of it, elbows on thighs, head down, back curved outward toward the resident, who opened the man's gown and cleaned his skin with a cold antiseptic. Still, the resident physician didn't speak a word. He just pushed the needle into the patient's back. Ask any woman who has had an epidural during childbirth—a spinal tap is tricky. The doctor is trying to get the needle between vertebrae, through the tough spinal membrane and into the narrow spinal canal. This is uncomfortable, possibly painful, and for many people, terrifying.

The resident fished the needle around a bit, but failed to get to the spot he needed. The patient held himself as still as possible as the resident pulled the needle out and handed it to an intern, the next most experienced person in the line. The intern pushed the needle, tried to angle it correctly, missed, and pulled out. He never spoke to the patient. The attempts continued down the line through the medical students—one after another, none of the future physicians speaking to the patient—until it was my turn. I took the needle from my classmate and moved to stand behind the man. He sat up and turned around to look at me. He asked, "Halee, is it going to be okay?"

6

I put my hand on his shoulder and said, "Yes, Dad—it's going to be okay."

The man was my father.

That moment in my third year of medical school more than twenty years ago captures everything I tried to be as a doctor—caring, compassionate, connected to my patients—and everything we need to do better as a medical community.

Yet, at the time, like the rest of my classmates, I was focused on learning the "how" of practicing medicine. Mostly, that meant the vital work of learning the science. There are tens of thousands, maybe millions, of ways the human body can break down—involving 10 major organs, 206 bones, 640 muscles, 100 million neurons, and more than 37 trillion cells—treatable with more than 1,300 medications and hundreds of different procedures. Thanks to advances in clinical understanding, the number of tests and screenings that physicians are required to perform has skyrocketed—and that's good news. Every one of those advances represents a victory for human ingenuity, a step forward for medicine. But it's a lot to learn: one physician in medical practice found that she juggled 550 separate patient decisions in the course of an average day.[5] It's a lot to learn.

All physicians will tell you that they've never felt more knowledgeable about the human body than the day they graduated from medical school. They'll also tell you that they've never been less knowledgeable about what it means to actually be a physician, what it really takes to care for patients and do the things necessary to make them well, than they are on graduation day. That's what it means to progress in the field: It's not unlike becoming a skilled pilot, or an experienced teacher.

As I look back on that moment today, my perspective is broader. I'm more focused on the "why." In that hospital room with my dad, we allowed ourselves to be too focused on the science, too disconnected from the fundamental reasons most of us went into medicine, the reasons I dreamed of being a physician from the age of eight: to heal and care for human beings.

If you talk with any patient, physician, or medical practice leader about the practice of medicine, you quickly realize that all three have the same thing in common: as much as they recognize the significance of the science of medicine and the importance of the business of medicine, the part of medicine that's most important to them is the human side—the big-hearted, patient-focused, high-touch, active-listening, caring, compassionate, empathetic part of medicine that has been at the heart of the doctor-patient relationship from the very beginning. For physicians, it is the place where experience, instinct, and passion for the skill of medicine converge. For patients, it is the home of care, connection, and communication—the things that make them feel valued, listened to, and cared for in moments of pain, fear, and vulnerability. For administrators, it's the place where value and impact can be seen and measured, where the sense of purpose and meaning that motivates them are found.

For over twenty-five hundred years, practitioners from the father of medicine, Hippocrates, to the father of modern medicine, William Osler, have described this part of health care as the *art of medicine*.

Sadly, today that art is on life support.

The art of medicine is being crowded out by the science of medicine—and its emphasis on evidence-based procedures, well-meaning protocols, and advances in Big-Health-Data-churning information technology. And it's being squeezed out by the business of medicine—and its focus on time-consuming but questionable quality metrics, endless billing procedures, and an adherence to process that doesn't necessarily put patients first. Put another way, the science and business of medicine have combined with a superficial focus on things like hospital gowns to essentially act like a Quentin Tarantino character going "medieval" on the art of medicine. But perhaps I understate.

New Kids on the Block

That analogy isn't meant to sound as harsh as it likely seems, because as brutally violent as Tarantino movies are, they are often fantastically told stories with significant meaning and social commentary. Asserting that the business and science of medicine have combined to push out the art of medicine is not meant to suggest that the two aren't vital. Quite the contrary. I, maybe like you, happen to revere the contributions that science has made to medicine. And I, perhaps also like you, really admire good business practices and the part they have played in funding research and developing new lifesaving equipment. As we will see in the following chapters, there is little question that the business and science of medicine are absolutely crucial to the effective practice of modern medicine. But in the same way that a chocolate chip cookie isn't as good if you remember the sugar and flour but forget the chocolate chips, the business and science of medicine without the art leave a lot—*a lot*—to be desired in American health care today.

As recently as two generations ago, this wasn't an issue because science and business didn't have a lot to offer. The role of science was largely in the background until the 1930s, when the discovery of penicillin ignited a new era of medical breakthroughs. Ever since, research, medications, and groundbreaking therapies have shifted what were traditionally thought of as untreatable illnesses and disease—like cancer, chronic lower respiratory disease, and heart disease, which are the three leading causes of mortality in the United States—into manageable chronic conditions. As data analytics, superfast computers, digital technology, and other breakthroughs enabled by science play a bigger and bigger role in informing medical decision-making, science has carved out a new and powerful role as the steadfast partner of the business of medicine—which is also enjoying a new day in the sun.

It may surprise some people to learn that the business of medicine is not a twenty-first-century invention. Health care has always been a business, as far back as the days when Hippocrates and his peers practiced medicine. Whether it was three goats, a gold coin, or a bank note, some type of payment was typically exchanged for medical services, and institutions of government or learning funded research. However, since the 1970s, business has been the major force directing the *practice* of medicine. Together, the business and science of medicine are the new kids on the block—the bright, shiny new things.

Ideally, as I've suggested, the art, science, and business of medicine would work together in a harmonious partnership, each upholding the other and contributing all it has to offer to the whole. And sometimes (as we'll find in later chapters) this partnership works well. When it does, the results are magnificent for patients and doctors, not to mention for scientists and investors.

However, as science and business have risen in significance and strength, too often their combined actions within medicine serve only to overpower, devalue, and squeeze out the art of medicine. This problem is showing up in ways that are making patients, physicians, and medical practice administrators miserable, while throwing out of balance our national aspirations for better population health at decreasing cost. It's leading to a potentially historic generation-long crisis in health care at precisely the moment when Americans can least afford it either personally or as a nation.

Patients, physicians, and medical practices are all fed up with the things that interfere with the relationship and care between doctor and patient: from the thirteen-minute visits consumed by doctors staring at computer screens, to endless referrals and networks where nobody seems to be in charge of care, to confusion about bills and insurance plans and deductibles.

There is no question that science and business are essential in our $3 trillion-plus health-care industry. But that doesn't mean we should sit back and stay silent as both overstep their bounds. The first step to solving a problem is admitting that you have one: The science and business of medicine have conspired to prioritize the very things that drive physicians and patients as far apart as two middle schoolers who asked the same girl to the school dance. We've reached the point where the average physician now spends nearly two hours on paperwork[6] for every hour spent with patients, if they're lucky. In fact, one study found that internal medicine interns actually spend just 12 percent of their time with patients and 40 percent on computer-related tasks.[7]

In fact, when I look back on that experience with my father nearly twenty-five years ago, I now recognize that my generation of physicians was on the leading edge of a trend that has changed medicine, mostly for the worst.

The Doctor Is Out

As anybody frustrated by our health-care system today knows, this loss of balance between art, science, and business in medicine has had a profound effect on patients' experience. Under the headline "In America, the Art of Doctoring Is Dying," physician and memoirist Jerald Winakur summed up his four-decade career in internal medicine and geriatrics with this 2016 lament in *The Washington Post*:

> There is no doubt that the kind of medicine I was fortunate to practice is disappearing.... Young primary-care doctors are relegated to assembly-line clinics; their patients pass through as widgets, not as individuals with complex inner lives, wrought family structures, varied spiritual and cultural beliefs—not to mention their individual capacities to understand and deal with their medical symptoms, diagnoses and multiple medications, as well as their own hopes and fears. Physicians are now insulated from knowing too much about their patients. It is all about the technology, the testing, the imaging, the electronic health record, the data—once collected by the doctor, but now so regulated and overwhelming that paramedical professionals have been enlisted to record the so-called minutiae, the often rote information in which may lie important clues. Some of

these may remain forever buried, the patient not wanting to share sensitive details with just anyone, especially someone who no longer makes eye contact, whose face remains buried behind a computer screen, who seems uninterested or just unskilled in reading body language—that downward glance, that shift in the chair, that half-swallowed response.[8]

As we will see later, it's possible to go overboard and wish for the days when art and art alone ruled medicine, like when dinosaurs ruled the earth, which also isn't helpful. But there probably isn't a single patient, doctor, or medical practice in America that doesn't identify with Dr. Winakur's words at some level. This is the exact conversation I have with my husband every night when he comes home from his pediatric practice. It's what I talk about with friends and fellow physicians over drinks before we discuss work gossip, the latest political scandal, or our families. In fact, in every corner of this country, whenever three or more medical professionals get together—over lunch, on break, after hours, during rounds, at nurse's stations, even in the operating room—we commiserate over the loss of art.

Here's what physicians know to be true: In prioritizing business and science over art in medicine, we are making it much harder to build the trust between patients and physicians necessary to bring about the improved results, better quality, and lower costs we all want in health care today. Studies confirm what instinct has told us from the very beginning: When doctors have the time to do what's necessary with their patients—look patients in the eye, listen to them, learn from them, lay hands on them, empathize with them, communicate with them, give trust, and earn trust—patients are much more likely to take the steps necessary to get healthy or stay healthy. When the art of medicine isn't present, everything in health care becomes more of an uphill fight.

Which isn't to say that art's champions have come out looking for a fight. No matter how exalted they are in their specialty or field of expertise, nearly all medical professionals have responded to the overreach of the science and business of medicine at the expense of its art with such disengagement that it threatens to undermine the ability of physicians to be effective advocates for patients. Indeed, a massive 2012 survey by the Physicians Foundation found that 82 percent of physicians believe they have "little ability to change the health care system."[9] Tragically, this is also one of the many reasons one in three young doctors today exhibit symptoms of clinical depression, and why the 2016 Physicians Foundation report found that half of the 17,000 respondents to its survey wouldn't recommend medicine as a profession.[10]

People go into medicine with a desire to be of help to others; medicine is a calling, one of the highest and best aspirations that exist in this world. It sounds a little pathetic to say it out loud, but after completing medical school, too many of those who started out with high ideals end up feeling like M.D. stands for "miserable doctor." The misery stems in large part from the very ways in which the business and science of medicine are overstepping their bounds, crowding out the primary reason most medical professionals entered the field—and, it needs to be said, went way into debt in the process—at the expense of effective patient care. Somehow we have managed to turn the most promising moment in the 2,500-year history of medicine into the most discouraging moment in the 250-year history of American health care.

And all the pretty hospital gowns in the world, while sure-fire crowd-pleasers, aren't going to bring health care back into balance.

When Art Disappears

This is the sleeper issue that too few people are talking about, the real reason for the American health-care crisis that lurks right around the corner: An entire generation of doctors in their thirties, forties, and fifties is disenchanted with their profession in ways that could have severe consequences for the long-term health of America. Not because they're at retirement age, but because they

are tired of sacrificing the human side of medicine to the complicated bureaucratic hurdles, clerical demands, and regulatory con-
trols that are defining an ever-growing part of our health-care
system today.

Which is not to suggest malicious motives: At various times,
all of these burdens began with the noblest of intentions. Over the
past fifty years, conventional wisdom has stated that we should
use the insights of science and the levers of business to improve
health-care outcomes. Great ideas, but while we were on the way
to achieving our stellar goals, nobody thought to look holistically at
the totality of all of new pressures being brought to bear on the system's delicate balance. Today there are so many mandates, directives, regulations, and penalties overwhelming physicians, medical
practices, and even patients that their joint ability to leverage their
knowledge, empathy, and expertise gets treated as an afterthought.

As the balance shifts, evidence shows what hardly comes as
news to the people who pass in and out of America's health-care
system every day: Patients are the ones who pay the highest price—
in the form of longer wait times, greater hassles, endless paperwork, more runaround, more confusion, increased medical errors,
and layer upon layer of issues that keep creating greater distance
between patients and their doctors. And with America adding the
equivalent of a pro football stadium full of baby boomer retirees
every single week until 2030—all of whom are entering their most
health-care-dependent years—the fun is just getting started.

Here's the real irony: The human side of medicine—the compassion, communication, and empathy that lie at the heart of the art of
medicine—is essential to achieving the outcomes that matter most
to the business and science sides of medicine.

Within health care, there has been an unyielding assumption
embedded in both the protocols of science and the metrics of business: that patients will comply with what their doctors ask them to
do. This is why balance matters: Study after study has shown that
when the art of medicine disappears, there's a significant and neg-

ative impact on health. When patients don't feel valued and heard as human beings, their overall sense of well-being and willingness to trust the system will suffer. And then they're much less likely to follow the steps that can help them manage their diabetes, lose weight, or deal with whatever their specific health challenge may be. If patients don't feel a connection to their doctors when problems come up, they are less likely to seek help until those problems become much worse and more expensive. In other words, in losing the art of medicine, we're sabotaging the broader goals we hold for America's health-care system.

Back to Balance:
The Art, Science, and Business of Medicine

What is the answer? We need to bring the art, science, and business of medicine back into balance—with each side playing its part and no more to drive the healthy outcomes that we all desire from health care today.

Rebalancing the health-care system isn't going to be easy, as I know full well. For the past twenty-five years, I've been a practicing pediatrician, the spouse of a physician, the owner of a medical practice, a practice leader, a hospital executive, a chief medical officer, a business consultant, the wife of a cancer survivor, and the daughter of a chronically ill father. I've seen every hard, messy, and mystifying challenge our health-care system has to offer. I know what it means to negotiate contracts on behalf of nearly a thousand physicians and what it takes to remove more than a dozen Trix stuck up a child's nose. I have felt the fear and sense of helplessness that comes with thinking I'm going to lose both my father and my husband to terrible diseases, and I have known the fury that comes when another administrator asks me to fill out another form covering exactly the same material I filled out five minutes before. I know how it feels to go cross-eyed looking through thousands of medical codes at midnight, to spend decades paying off medical school debt (still not done!), and to argue with an insurance company for two hours on the phone to get a simple liver function test approved. I also know how it feels to save a life—and what it feels like to lose six young patients in a single night.

Today, as the CEO of an organization that represents 40,000 practice administrators and executives in 18,000 health-care organizations across all fifty states, where more than 400,000 physicians practice, providing close to 50 percent of the health care in the United States, I know it doesn't have to be this way. I wrote this book because I want the country that helped the world cure polio and transplant a human heart and tame a virus as deadly as HIV to stop thinking that we should somehow settle for mediocrity in our health-care system and instead believe that we can achieve excellence once again. I know we can do it because I've seen it: In every part of America today, there are medical practices that are providing a glimpse at a better path forward—people who are asking the right questions, focusing on the right priorities, achieving the desired results, and proving that we can bring health care back into balance to benefit all of us. You will meet some of them in this book

What this movement back to balance is proving is that change doesn't happen from the top down; it actually works much better from the bottom up. Solving the challenges laid out in this book won't require a lot more time and money to make health care what it should be: more patient-centered, more rewarding, more engaging, and more sustainable. But what it will take is a focus on healthier people rather than a focus on disease; a system where art, science, and business work together to enable people to do what is right for each patient, with the time and resources to address more than just the basics; and with providers—doctors, nurses, medical practice staff—who feel supported in their drive to do their best work to help patients be as healthy as possible.

In the chapters that follow, I invite you to join me on a journey through the many surprising, appalling, inspiring, poignant, hair-raising, and ridiculously funny territories within which medicine lives today. Along the way, I hope to point out features of the art, the science, and the business of medicine, to bring them more clearly into view. You'll learn what dinosaurs have to do with the art of medicine and what customized sneakers have to do with the science. You may be surprised to hear that the most profound insight on health care in the twenty-first century was uttered by a twentieth-century film character: Buckaroo Banzai. You'll learn which South Park character has apparently gone to work for the federal government and which of Carrie Bradshaw's advice columns on *Sex and the City* health care is shamelessly violating today. You'll learn the three questions to ask at the practice level that can help define what balance means for you, and the five paradigm shifts at the macro level that can help start a new conversation.

My goal is to be part of activating a movement to bring balance back to the art, science, and business of medicine, so that each of us—no matter who we are and what we do—can respond to our own highest calling and help one another expect more and get more out of health care in our lives.

As Hippocrates put it twenty-five centuries ago: "Where there is love of man, there is also love of the art. For some patients, though conscious that their position is perilous, recover their health simply through their contentment with the physician." Yes, making hospital gowns that protect our backsides along with our dignity is an important step to improving health care in America today. But restoring the fundamental relationship of trust between patients and physicians is a much more important step.

This is a book about why it is up to us to bring balance back to the art, science, and business of medicine and how we can make health care work as well in practice as in promise.

CHAPTER 2

Just Because We Can, Does It Mean We Should?

What do dinosaurs, George Clooney,
and the art of medicine have
in common?

IN OCTOBER OF 1989, two men had lunch together at a Hollywood restaurant. Neither could have guessed the mammoth impact their discussion that day would have on popular culture for decades to follow. Their names might give you a hint of what happened: I'm talking about Michael Crichton and Steven Spielberg.

It's easy to get giddy imagining the conversation between them. Crichton was a Harvard Medical School graduate who'd become a mega-bestselling novelist and sought-after screenwriter. Spielberg was the most celebrated film director of his generation, a creative visionary who had changed the way movies were made.

The two men had known each other since 1970. Back then, Universal Studios had just bought the film rights to Crichton's novel *The Andromeda Strain*, a fast-paced thriller about a team of scientists trying to save the planet from an alien microorganism that had hopped a ride to Earth on a military satellite. Universal invited the author to visit the facility, and his tour guide that day was a rising star who had just become the youngest director ever to sign a seven-year contract with a major Hollywood studio: Spielberg. The two discovered a mutual affection for telling human stories about the dangers posed by overreliance on science and technology.

Fast-forward to 1989. During their lunch on this momentous day, Spielberg and Crichton started out discussing a screenplay Crichton had written called *Code Blue*, a medical drama based on his experiences as a Harvard student, back when he still believed he wanted to be a doctor. Spielberg loved the script and committed to directing it—but then asked Crichton about other projects he might have in the hopper. The author gave a cagey answer: He was putting the finishing touches on a secret project he didn't want to talk about.

Spielberg was far too intrigued to let it go at that. And Crichton relented but swore Spielberg to secrecy before fessing up that his next book was about "dinosaurs and DNA." Those words got Spielberg absolutely hooked—he was already sure he wanted to direct the film. But he needed to know more.[11]

Weeks of prodding later, Crichton confided to Spielberg that the story was about a remote island amusement park featuring living dinosaurs! In his novel, geneticists extract the DNA of actual dinosaurs from mosquitoes trapped in amber, and use that DNA to recreate ancient life-forms for the amusement of tourists in today's world. Visitors to the park interact with the dinosaurs—see a brontosaurus casually eating a tree, walk past a sleeping *T. rex*, experience velociraptors that hunt in packs—and then something goes horribly, horribly wrong.

By the time Crichton had finished telling the story, not only did Spielberg commit to directing the film, but the two men had agreed to pursue the dinosaur movie ahead of the medical film.

Crichton published *Jurassic Park* the next year, and in 1993, the film version of the book by the same name became a worldwide phenomenon, grossing more than $1 billion and launching a popular franchise still going strong. After that, Crichton and Spielberg adopted the *Code Blue* script for television, and that medical drama, renamed *ER*, went on to become widely celebrated, running for fifteen years and catapulting its headliner—George Clooney—to megastardom.

When Crichton was later asked about his favorite part of the movie *Jurassic Park*, he zeroed in on a line spoken by actor Jeff Goldblum's character, who watched the now-escaped dinosaurs wreak havoc on the humans occupying the island. Goldblum's character—whose tall, chaos-theory-spouting intellectual was a stand-in for the six-nine author—said to the founders of Jurassic Park, "Your scientists were so preoccupied with whether or not they *could* that they didn't stop to think if they *should*."

Those familiar with Crichton's career can recognize the theme at work in this sentence. Again and again through eighteen blockbuster novels—thirteen of which were made into major films—Crichton had a lot to say about the loss of art and humanity in the face of science, technology, and business. As society moved at a breakneck pace to pry open the long-hidden mysteries of science, Crichton stood astride history time and time again and asked: Are we asking the right questions? Are we framing choices in the right way? Are we aware of the dangers we may unlock at the end of a journey, or are we so focused on the rush of discovery that we're blinded to where it may lead?

Just because we *can*, does that mean we *should*?

Michael Crichton never asked these questions more passionately or with more authority than he did about health care. Although he never practiced medicine, the first nonfiction book he wrote was about the years he spent as a Harvard medical student interning at Massachusetts General Hospital in Boston. Published in 1970, *Five Patients* is a cautionary tale. It points to the way that the art of medicine was being challenged for the first time in history by the science and business of medicine. Dr. Crichton hit a nerve that's just as poignant today as it was during the Vietnam War era in which it was written.

In the years since *Five Patients* was released, two things have shaped the way we discuss health care. First, the practice of medicine is now controlled by science and business. Second, there are widespread laments by patients and health-care providers alike about the loss of the art of medicine, and how that loss is felt from both sides of the stethoscope—from patients who complain that physicians no longer have time to listen to them, learn from them, fully explain complicated medicine, and treat them with compassion; and from doctors who complain about having to rush from appointment to appointment, interact with computer screens more than patients, and deal with hassles from insurance companies and regulators at the expense of effective clinical care. As the chapters of this book unfold, the way in which these two things are directly related will become clear.

If he were here today (sadly, we lost him to cancer in 2008), I think Michael Crichton would be the first to say that we aren't asking the right questions in medicine anymore—and because we aren't asking the right questions, we're not achieving our goals. The questions we ask ourselves matter. Instead of asking, "How do we apply more science and business to develop the best processes?" we need to ask ourselves, "How do we get to what we really want: happier patients, lower cost, and better-quality medicine? What is missing from the current picture that is preventing us from achieving what we want to achieve?"

While many in health care believe that the solution to high costs and poor outcomes is yet more reliance on science and business, that's not what we are missing today: We are missing the art of medicine. We should be working toward the balance between art, science, and business that will free doctors and medical practices to give patients the quality personal care they want and expect.

Much like the book *Jurassic Park*, where DNA trapped in amber is used to bring dinosaurs into creation by people blissfully and arrogantly unaware of the unforeseen consequence of their actions— we are engineering a similar situation in health care. The more we try to dictate the behavior of healers with dozens upon dozens of directives and protocols that seek to define in minute detail every second of the interaction between patients and physicians—each written without awareness of, and often in direct conflict to, the other directives—the more we turn what has been the most human part of medicine into something unnatural and overbearing, with catastrophic results. The problem is, even while we try to manufacture outcomes, human nature remains largely unchanged. All the science and business in the world won't change the fact that if human beings are going to follow the advice of their doctors, they've got to feel listened to, understood, and cared for. As the revered doctor and educator Francis Weld Peabody wrote nearly a century ago, "The significance of the intimate personal relationship between physician and patient cannot be too strongly emphasized, for in an extraordinarily large number of cases, both diagnosis and treatment are directly dependent on it. The secret to the care of the patient ... is in caring for the patient."[12] By diminishing the human connection, we are throwing medicine out of equilibrium, while allowing the science and business of medicine to rise up like those intelligent velociraptors in Crichton's novel.

And when medicine is reduced to only business and science, it sets up a great nesting ground for hatching velociraptors that grow up to hunt in packs. If instead the art of medicine is given its due and a balance is struck with science and business, we experience the highest and best that medical practice can offer.

The Surprising Thing About Surprising Things

I grew up watching reruns of *Marcus Welby, M.D.* with my mom. Welby was the friendly family doctor who had learned everyone's names, treated families throughout their lives, and knew individuals as people, not just patients. What I rarely saw was Marcus Welby making difficult medical decisions based on the latest scientific research or sending a bill after his services were performed.

And I never ever saw Marcus Welby:

- dealing with a patient by telling him which drug they needed based on an ad they'd seen on TV

- sitting with eyes glued to a computer screen six feet away from his patient
- turning patients away because he didn't accept their insurance
- filling out reports for federal agencies to document his productivity
- fielding questions from unhappy patients who had looked up Welby's advice on WebMD and decided he must be wrong

Too often when people speak of the art of medicine, it's with hollow reverence for this kind of ideal, downplaying the role of science, while sneering in disdain at the role of business.

This Marcus Welby image of a bygone day might give us warm and tingly feelings, but it never was the ideal: Doctors have never practiced art for art's sake only, nor should we kid ourselves that such an ideal is worth pursuing. In every previous era, the art of medicine has always existed within the context of the science and business of medicine. Many times the art was more vital simply because for most of history neither science nor business had much to offer. As Crichton himself once wrote, if you charted scientific discovery and business breakthroughs during the 2,500-year history of medicine, you'd see a very long, flat line with a slight tick upward in the middle of the nineteenth century, and then a sharp jump after the discovery and commercialization of penicillin in the middle of the twentieth century—when our modern era began to come into view.

This is the surprising thing about surprising things: The art of medicine is valuable *within the context* of science, *informed by* business. None of us want to go back to a time when science and business were both so flimsy. We want to go forward, embracing the extraordinary benefits of science and business while balancing them with the things that only the art of medicine can provide—the fine-tuned experience, the integration of personal understanding and compassion that *enables us to build the trust necessary* to generate the outcomes we want as a nation. It's in the balance of art, science, and business that we find the best and highest practice of medicine.

What does that balance look like to me? Whenever I'm asked why I became a physician, what comes to mind is the face of one of my patients, a bright young girl who liked to ask "Why?" about everything I did. We'll call her Brittany.

On a Friday afternoon just a few years after I began practicing as a pediatrician, I received a call from a caseworker at the Women, Infants, and Children program. WIC, as it's known, is a federal program that provides nutritious food, maternal support, and health referrals to low-income children and their families. WIC monitors every child in the program for iron deficiency, among other things. The week before, five-year-old Brittany had come in with her mother for a required blood test.

"I am calling to inform you," the WIC case manager casually said, "that her hemoglobin is 4."

"Is that a mistake?" I asked, stunned.

"We don't know, but we're obligated to call you and let you know."

Hemoglobin is a protein in red blood cells that attaches itself to oxygen as blood passes through the lungs and helps carry the oxygen to tissues throughout the body. A normal hemoglobin level is 16 or 17. A result of 4 is intensely worrisome, especially in a child, because it means the body is being starved of the oxygen it needs to thrive.

I hung up and immediately called Brittany's mom, whom we'll call Amanda, at her job. "I need you to bring Brittany in. I'm not comfortable waiting until Monday to see her." They took the bus to my office.

When I walked into the exam room to see them, I couldn't believe the change in Brittany from the week before. She looked sick, pale, and drawn—and didn't have the energy to ask me a single question as I examined her, representative of the kind of extreme fatigue associated with extremely low blood counts. Her heart rate was up and her liver and spleen were enlarged.

I took Amanda into the hall. "Look, Amanda, Brittany has something serious going on. I'm sorry to have to say this, but I think it may be leukemia. I can't let you go home without knowing for sure. We'll know more soon. I'm going to give you a referral for her because I don't have the tools here to tell you exactly what's wrong."

I called my friend, a children's cancer doctor and blood specialist. "I need to ask you a favor, I need you to see her today. I know it's four-thirty on a Friday, but I'm sure this kid has leukemia." My friend is a wonderful doctor and an outstanding human being, and gave the response I expected: "Of course."

"I'm going to draw blood here and send it with her so you don't need to poke her twice. What do you need?"

She described various tubes and colors—purple top, red top, tiger top, etc. I took notes, hung up, and returned to Amanda and Brittany. "I'm sending you to my friend's office, and she'll figure out what's happening." We drew the blood—Brittany barely made a peep—and then I taped the little bag full of tubes to her shirt so they wouldn't get mislaid.

Meanwhile, Amanda had called a family member to drive them to the doctor's office. And it wasn't just Brittany who needed empathy and care that day. Naturally, this young mom was both nervous and scared, and looked to me to be a calming presence. I let Amanda know that I understood her worries and reassured her that her daughter would be in excellent hands.

They left, and I waited. About ninety minutes later, my friend called me. "She *does* have leukemia. But we'll take care of her. She's going to do great."

Today Brittany *is* doing great. She's in her late teens and is more concerned with Instagram likes than her past medical history. My friend still sees her occasionally for checkups. Many times in the years that have passed since then, I have wondered what would have happened if someone who didn't have my education, experience, and trusting relationship with Brittany's mom had answered that call.

As long as human beings like Brittany or Amanda have sought to be healed or comforted by other human beings, the practice of medicine has been comprised of three parts: the business of medicine (how we pay), the science of medicine (how we treat), and the art of medicine (how we care). Medical students are taught a quotation from the father of modern medicine, Sir William Osler, who wrote in his book *Aequanimitas* in 1904, "The practice of medicine is an art, not a trade; a calling, not a business; a calling in which your heart will be exercised equally with your head." And then in one of the most-quoted lines in the history of health care, he added, "The practice of medicine is an art, *based on* science."

That line has been quoted in more than a dozen books over the past two decades, often by those who look starry-eyed at the art of medicine. But I seriously doubt that Osler would say the same thing today. Illness and diseases that routinely killed people in their thirties and forties when Dr. Osler was alive are now manageable chronic conditions. The magnificent discoveries from the frontiers of science that allow us to live longer and with a higher quality of life all prove that modern medicine is based on a solid foundation of science.

The successes brought about by scientific understanding should not be celebrated irrespective of the value of the art, and yet despite 2,500 years (at least) of scholarship about the art of medicine, that art has fallen from favor.

Brittany's story illustrates why art is so important.

At the heart of a physician's ability to effectively listen, diagnose, treat, and heal a patient is a timeless covenant: the covenant of trust. In 2004, physician Alice K. Jacobs argued in a keynote address to the American Heart Association: "Trust is essential to patients, in their willingness to seek care, their willingness to reveal sensitive information, their willingness to submit to treatment, and their willingness to follow recommendations. They must be *willing* for us to be *able*."[13]

The reason Amanda, Brittany's mom, was willing to take my

call at work, and then immediately leave work to bring Brittany into my office, was because she *trusted* me to tell her the truth and to do the right thing for her and her daughter. We already had a doctor-patient relationship built on clear and true communication. She accepted it when I told her that Brittany likely had leukemia because she *trusted* my judgment and knew I would never bring up such a diagnosis unless I believed it was important to her child's life. And she went to the office of a doctor she had never met before because she *trusted* me to send her to someone who would have the same level of care and compassion for her daughter that I did.

A mountain of research supports the link between trust and good results for patients. A review of clinical trials published in *Health Affairs* in 2015 revealed that a trusting relationship between physicians and patients based on compassion, empathy, and good communication can have a profound effect on patient health. Trust aids efforts to control diabetes, lower cholesterol, and control pain. Trust improves the physical and mental quality of life for cancer patients. Trust encourages people to get regular preventive care. Trust gives older patients better outcomes and more long-lasting independence. Relationships built on trust have been shown to reduce anxiety, depression, post-traumatic stress disorder, and a patient's use of intensive care at the end of life. These relationships are linked not only to lower hospital readmission rates for heart failure and pneumonia but also to more successful treatment regimens, lower health-care costs, and much higher patient satisfaction scores.[14]

I happily acknowledge that Brittany's story isn't just about the art of medicine. It also illustrates that the highest and best practice of the art of medicine requires the integration of business and science as well. I wouldn't have suspected leukemia if I didn't know the pathology, nor would my friend have been able to successfully treat it. (Thank you, science of medicine.) And if there hadn't been health insurance—in this case, paid by taxpayers through the Medicaid program—what would have covered the years of treatment Brittany received? (Thank you, business of medicine.)

This, then, is the dilemma at the heart of health care today. For America to achieve the ambitious national goals it has set to reduce costs, increase quality, and improve results in medicine, trust between physicians and patients, as embodied in the art of medicine, is absolutely essential—because if it's absent, patients won't do the things necessary to achieve those goals. Yet every policy, prescription, and medical practice mandate that has been put forward the past forty years has served to advance or advantage the science and business of medicine at the unanticipated expense of medicine. In the process, a thousand tiny and not-so-tiny wedges have been driven between patients, physicians, and medical practice administrators while pushing them further and further apart. (We'll get more into the details of how this is happening in later chapters.)

And it shows. A 2014 study by the Harvard School of Public Health in Boston found that Americans' trust in the medical profession has nose-dived: just 34 percent of U.S. adults polled said they had "great confidence in the leaders of the medical profession," down from 76 percent in 1966.[15] It's a problem that is more pronounced in America than in any other developed country: The same survey found that the United States ranks twenty-fourth of twenty-nine countries in the public trust of physicians. Fewer than six in ten Americans are willing to agree that doctors in the United States can be trusted—falling far behind top-ranked Switzerland, where doctors are trusted by more than eight in ten. Americans are more inclined than the people of almost every other nation to say that their country's medical personnel are motivated by factors other than better public health—including personal gain.

It's not just patients who are clamoring for strong relationships that build trust. Physicians are, too. When more than 17,000 physicians were asked in a wide-ranging 2016 survey on the state of the medical profession what they found most satisfying about the practice of medicine, an overwhelming 73.8 percent said it was this relationship between doctors and patients.[16] Yet nearly three out of every four of those same doctors said that outside factors severely affected their ability to provide quality care to their patients. Succinctly put, the art of medicine is vital to building trust in medicine.

Moving away from the art opens an abyss separating us from what matters most in medicine—for patients, physicians, and medical practice administrators alike—while simultaneously keeping us from the very things we need to achieve the results we all want.

How do we change that? We start with the art.

The Gargoyle That Is Medicine Without Art

The first time I was in Paris, it was part of an eight-country, seven-day bus tour of Europe. At an exhibit in the Louvre, I remember seeing something so disturbing it has stayed with me for the past thirty-five years.

It was called Art Grotesque.

The exhibition featured pieces of art that put the term "ugly cry" into relief. It took sculptures of people and twisted and contorted them into horribly unnerving shapes. Think of a skull coming out of the open mouth of a skull, its own mouth open, revealing smaller and then smaller skulls. Imagine a pig with the torso of an overweight man where the head should be, the figure wearing a garment made of gold coins and decked in shining jewels. That display, seen in beautiful pink Parisian light, haunts my nightmares still.

Those images often come to me when I think of the science and business of medicine being practiced without the art. It is indeed art grotesque. It is medicine stripped of humanity. And for every miraculous save in medicine, there are tales of what happens when medicine is practiced without the art, without relationship or soul—when physicians don't see a patient as a person but as a collection of symptoms.

Some doctors have even experienced this as patients themselves.

In the late summer of 2016, Eric Topol, a cardiologist and professor of genomics at California's Scripps Research Institute, finally decided to become one of 750,000 Americans each year who have knee replacement surgery.

Since he was a teenager, Topol had suffered with bad knees, caused by a rare condition known as osteochondritis dissecans that caused his knees to dislocate frequently. He had surgery at age twenty that made his condition bearable over the next four decades, but as he grew older, the pain forced Topol to give up one thing after another that he loved: running, then hiking, then tennis. Eventually, anti-inflammatory medications weren't enough, so he received steroid injections directly into his knee joint. When that didn't work anymore, he had no choice but to get a new knee. His orthopedist told him that he was a perfect candidate, and that the only potential danger was an infection, which happened very rarely.

As Topol described it later in *The Washington Post*, the surgery went well, and the orthopedist started him immediately on intense physical therapy, to create the widest possible range of motion before scar tissue set in—first with home sessions, and then at a popular facility his orthopedist recommended.[17] The standard protocol was applied. The PT staff even gave him preprinted sheets that outlined the daily home exercises he would need to do.

But from the moment physical therapy began, Topol was in agony beyond the scope of painkillers. Four weeks after his surgery, he wasn't getting better, so his orthopedist prescribed eight more weeks of intensive hour-long sessions, three times weekly, with an equal amount of torture at home. At some point the knee turned purple. It swelled. It stiffened. It hurt so badly that Topol had crying fits. He couldn't sleep. He was getting desperate, turning to alternative treatments. Nothing helped. His doctor suggested that if he just waited a year, the swelling would go down, and the scar tissue could be removed.

Then a friend recommended another physical therapist, one who had more than forty years of experience under her belt. Though skeptical, Topol went. The therapist didn't exercise his knee. Instead, she started by asking him a lot of questions. She took a detailed history of his health. She asked about surgeries when he was a teenager. She asked about medical procedures from years before, for problems that had nothing to do with his knee.

After they had talked for nearly an hour, she led him through a round of questioning about a frozen shoulder he'd had five years before. It didn't seem like anything on its face, but when viewed through the lens of his osteochondritis dissecans, the information she gathered about his shoulder told her that he had a much higher likelihood than normal of getting painful scarring in his joints.

She then turned to a physical exam—not forcing him to exercise, but instead evaluating his bloated knee. She immediately ordered him to stop the torturous weights and exercises and gave him a customized workout plan, along with anti-inflammatory medication. She told him that if he'd seen her the day after his surgery, she would have recommended this approach from the start, and never once would have let him pursue the plan called for in the treatment protocols. What struck him the most was a full page of instructions that the physical therapist wrote by hand—not a preprinted sheet, but a customized protocol tailored to his personal situation.

It was like night and day. Within a few days, the swelling went down. The discoloration and pain went away. Every few days, the PT texted him asking about "our knee." As he improved, she added further gentle exercises to his regimen. After three months of misery, Topol felt rescued.

When asked later what saved him, he described the art of medicine in a harmonious dance with science and business. An experienced medical professional was willing to treat him as a person and find out what was different about him (art). She then used her scientific knowledge to prescribe a course of treatment unique to his circumstances (science). He also felt lucky that his health insurance paid for much of it (business).

Topol elaborated on how his physical therapist's practice of the art of medicine had brought the other two into balance. The biggest problem, he said, was that he "was suffering from one-size-fits-all medicine." (Science without art.) The answer, he wrote, was that "the patient, in fact, has to be understood as a unique human being."

Not every physical therapist would guess that a rare complication would derail standardized therapy before therapy even began, but a surprising number of experienced medical professionals who follow their guts show a high success rate over time. Their art, based on their experience and expertise, greatly benefits their patients.

The art of medicine provides an intangible gestalt, a constellation of experiential moments that bestow a kind of intuition—a way of putting things together, things that at first might appear unrelated or irrelevant. This takes time to develop, and recognizing and understanding hidden patterns requires time as well. And the mere suggestion that a medical doctor could be consulting this kind of intuition tends to drive the rationalist, science-only minds in medicine straight out of their gourds. For to them, the idea that often there are answers the data won't suggest seems counterintuitive, but every single medical professional know it's true.

It's false to suggest that advocating for the art of medicine means denying the importance of science or business in medicine. It's not an either-or situation—we need a balance of all three. To deny the art of medicine is to deny human nature—something that has changed a lot less over the last 2,500 years than science and business have. As human beings, we are hardwired for human contact. Empathy and compassion are still important to us.

Picture someone in great pain and having trouble walking. Although "Angie" is only fifty-four, her joints are breaking down. X-rays reveal she's due for a double hip replacement. A surgeon with excellent ratings is accepted by her insurance. So far, so good.

Angie calls his office, and that's when things go bad. She wants an appointment to meet with the surgeon who will perform a complicated, fairly brutal surgery. "No," she's told by his office staff, "if you insist on meeting him beforehand, you'll delay your surgery. Just book it and he'll fix your joints. It's not as if you need to be friends."

Angie, like many other humans, is hardwired to feel the need to gain a sense of the man behind the surgeon's mask before going under his knife. She wants to trust him, wants a face-to-face meeting where she can get a personal experience of who he is. And now she begins to wonder why his office doesn't seem to understand. Is the surgeon a bad person? Does she really want him to be the one to be, in her words, "carving me up"? She's so undone by the cold and clinical way she's being treated that she feels hopeless and alone, completely at a loss for where to turn.

As Angie and countless others are discovering, medicine without art is scary and uncomfortable. Pain gets worse, fears and anxiety spiral, and treatments get delayed. As a society, we end up dealing with the fallout as complications increase. Costs actually go up because people wait until they're even sicker to finally seek the help they need. The consequences range from inconvenient to catastrophic.

Medicine without art is grotesque indeed.

I freely acknowledge that science and technology have changed all our lives, mostly for the better. Still, I don't want a computer to tell me I have cancer. I want a human—a human with experience, knowledge, and compassion—to reassure me and let me know what can be done. I doubt that anybody—at least anybody yet—wants a health-care system in which, as futurist Vinod Khosla describes it, "much of what physicians do—like checkups, testing, diagnosis, prescription, and behavior modification" are performed "by sensors, passive and active data collection, and analytics." I love the droids from *Star Wars* as much as anyone, but I'm not ready to disrobe in front of them and have them conduct my annual physical exam sans human contact—and neither are most Americans.

Contrary to our digital transformation, studies show that what patients want most from their health care is basic human connection: physicians who are caring and compassionate, who take the time to look them in the eye, who listen to them without interrupting, and who explain patiently until they understand.

All In:
The Case for Balance

There are days when it appears that the art, science, and business of medicine are vying for supremacy in a boxing ring instead of partnering on the dance floor. As I'll explain in later chapters, the interactions between them have become downright hostile at times, and if they continue to face off the way they are now, I'm afraid it's the patient who will end up getting knocked out.

As America struggles to find its way on health care, a welcome voice was scheduled to join the debate again in 2017. Nearly a decade after his death, an unpublished novel from Michael Crichton called *Dragon Teeth* would see its debut. Even from beyond the grave, Crichton still has the magic touch: National Geographic optioned the story for a six-part series, written by acclaimed screenwriter Graham Yost, famous for his work on the classic TV series *Band of Brothers,* produced by Steven Spielberg and Tom Hanks.

Dragon Teeth tells the story of Edward Drinker Cope and Othniel Charles Marsh, two of the great dinosaur hunters of the nineteenth century, in what Yost has described as "a big adventure story with science at its heart." The two men were fierce rivals during the so-called Bone Wars, a period of time after the Civil War in which the two former friends began scouring the American West to find dinosaur bones. Over the next thirty years, between them they would discover over 142 new species of dinosaurs (of which only thirty or so are valid today).

But the two men could not share the glory. Each wanted to be supreme; each cared only for promoting his own advantage at the expense of his rival. For more than two decades, Cope and Marsh engaged in escalating attacks and sabotages on the work of the other. Theirs was a zero-sum contest—a game in which the cumulative wins equal the cumulative losses—if there ever was one. In the end, the conflict left both of them financially ruined, publicly shamed, and physically in pain.

Cope was the first to die, in 1897, but not before trying to best Marsh one last time. On his deathbed, Cope issued a challenge, announcing that he was donating his skull to science for the purpose of having his brain measured, and asking Marsh to do the same. He maintained that he wanted to do this so posterity could record which of the two men had the bigger brain, and thus the greater intellect. Marsh never agreed. To this day, legend has it that Cope's skull is housed at the University of Pennsylvania.

Unlike the rivalry between Edward Drinker Cope and Othniel Charles Marsh, medicine is not all or nothing. Art and science and business are not in a zero-sum game. It's not about one achieving positive outcomes at the expense of the others. It's about finding and maintaining balance. It's about engaging excellence by doing what each of us does best, without diminishing what others do best. What we want overall is not art for art's sake, but art practiced in a solid partnership with business, and both on a foundation of science—so that all three together serve patients, providers, and the public.

That was Michael Crichton's message nearly fifty years ago. *Five Patients* was written at a moment of transition in the history of American health care from one era to another, from an age defined by art to the modern age defined more by science, technology, and business. Crichton saw this coming, too.

"It would thus appear," he wrote in 1970, "that all the functions of a doctor are being taken over either by other people or by machines. What will be left for the doctor of the future? Almost certainly he will begin to move in one of two directions. The first is clearly toward full-time research.... A second direction will be away from science toward the 'art' of medicine—the complex, very human problems of helping people adjust to disease processes; for there will always be a gap between the illnesses medicine faces and science's limitations in treating them. And there will always be a need for people to bridge that gap."[18]

There will always be a need for people to bridge that gap. Not either-or. Not zero-sum. But art in balance with business and science, focused on healing people.

CHAPTER 3

The People vs. The Patient

How science, data, and technology are
threatening the art of medicine.

ABOUT TEN YEARS AGO, I wanted to buy my husband Mike a special present for Christmas—something personal and thoughtful that would show my understanding of who he is. Good gift-giving is a point of pride for me, so I chose ... sneakers.

Sneakers might not seem like a particularly *special* gift to you, but these shoes—well, these were no off-the-rack, mass-produced, see-them-on-everybody's-feet shoes. They were custom-made personalized Chuck Taylor All Star High Tops from Converse—designed by me especially for Mike. Anyone who knows Mike will tell you that he is understated but always dependable, classic but always current, handsome but not at all showy, and as big a hit with older folks as he is with kids—in other words, Mike is the Chuck Taylor All Star High Tops of husbands. As soon as I discovered the site, I knew I had found the perfect opportunity to show how much I care.

With the choice of a casino-red (Mike's favorite color) upper body, I was off on a design odyssey spanning *twelve* different parts of the shoe. After the base color, I moved on to the heel stripe (navy blue), the laces (classic white), the eyelets (metallic silver). I chose sidewalls with a thin navy racing stripe running along the edge and near the sole and the logo (classic red, white, and blue). I even picked the color of the stitching used to sew the shoe together.

The next two choices made the shoes all Mike. For the lining,

I went with an Aztec red and white print in a geometric pattern of skulls (because he's a doctor) and all-seeing eyes (because he's got a bit of the mystic in him). The final option had me stumped initially, although it was the true reason behind the gift: I could have any word, phrase, or number I wanted embroidered on the outside of the shoe by the heel. His initials? Too preppy. Our wedding date? Definitely not. What would best represent my enigma of a husband?

I clicked in the field and typed crab poke—as in the Hawaiian fish salad. I'll leave out the why, because it's a story best left untold, but I knew what Mike would think of my phrase.

At that time, I could have ordered customized Nikes, Adidas, or Pumas. Today I can go to Chiko Shoes or Shoes of Prey and design a pair of heels or wedges or boots for myself. If I had the budget, I could do the same with a pair of Manolo Blahniks. More and more big brands are joining the custom-made shoe market every year. The ability to design our own footwear based on a refined set of options even has a catchy oxymoronic name: mass customization. Demand is so high, experts estimate the market at more than $2 billion. And according to the font of all modern knowledge, Wikipedia, it's the new frontier in business—although more than a decade ago, industry leaders in Europe studied it and then published the possibly overdramatized *Mass Customization and Footwear: Myth, Salvation or Reality?*[19]

When I bought Mike's shoes, I didn't realize I was part of the early growth of a new manufacturing movement. The idea of mass customization was first introduced in the mid-eighties, but the trend is reaching fever pitch today, and people love it. Of course social media and the rise in DIY have driven the trend, too. Younger generations are being taught the importance of "personal brand," of standing out and displaying who we are for all to see. Of course, the options available to me for each of those twelve parts of Mike's shoes weren't random. Converse chose them based on market analysis and data mining. It's not surprising that today, many of the options I picked for Mike have been replaced by other choices or given updated names. Tastes change.

The taste for customization, though, is only spreading. You can choose your own color blocks for leggings at Alala, add custom embroidery to your Levi's, and monogram just about any piece of clothing for a small fee. You can also personalize your M&Ms, your beer labels, your Swiss Army knife. And as it goes with many trends, the pornography industry has been at the forefront, or so I hear. (I'll leave you to do your own research on that.)

I can order the type of pillow I want in my room when I book a hotel, and if I'm a regular, I can register all my preferences with them and my room will be set up just as I like it when I arrive. A friend went to a "bespoke restaurant" for her anniversary. The maître d' called a couple of days beforehand and asked about likes and dislikes, not only for the husband and wife, but also for their guests. Then the chef made each of them a custom meal.

Every day we're asked how we want to receive communication, what news agencies we'd like in our feed, whether we want to use online scheduling to pick convenient appointments, and more. We can design how we interact and what we experience with businesses of all sizes. Companies feeding this appetite are smart, because once people get a taste of customized goods or adventures, they're hooked.

In almost every industry, research, data, and technological innovation are leading to higher personalization and more custom offerings. Big companies and small are using what they learn about their customers to cater to people's individual desires.

But somehow, with a few exceptions, the trend in health care seems to be the reverse, despite (or maybe because of) the pace of change and innovation when it comes to data and technology in medicine. People are increasingly being treated as if they're the same. Science and data are being used to *decrease* variability in an attempt to get doctors to treat patients in predictable ways. Now, predictability isn't necessarily a bad thing, but it can be when data is used to treat the disease and not the patient. Too often, data-driven health care means patients feel like numbers and doctors feel like ciphers beholden to pie charts.

When it comes to cures and treatments, the industry of medicine is shifting its focus to data sets. And those data sets are drawn from large segments of the population and then converted into treatment protocols based on averages. In a certain way, this makes sense: Today people's lives are longer, and they are living out those years with chronic illnesses. It makes sense to want to find out the best way to help them. And given that treating chronic disease is one of the biggest drivers of our national health-care budget, it makes sense that we want to try to reduce costs by finding the most efficient way to treat patients who suffer from them, and keep those patients from the extreme events that cause big spikes in costs.

Well, the methods and protocols that come about as a result of looking at data sets would work beautifully—if people were all alike. However, we're not. There isn't a one-size-fits-all diabetes patient or hypertension patient or heart disease patient, any more than there's a one-size-fits-all shoe.

This focus on data and technology leaves the art of medicine in a quandary. Doctors are expected to rely on data as opposed to what they learn about individual patients, and to treat individuals as data points rather than as people. But of course people cannot possibly conform individually to an average that's been derived from the population as a whole.

To be clear, I'm not here to malign science—far from it! I will never forget that on the front lines of medicine, the happy trifecta of research, data gathering, and technological innovation has brought us new cures, safer treatments, and better testing. Yet all of these exciting developments in medicine are being overshadowed by relentless statistical averaging, rigid protocols, and treatment by the numbers. For years now we have been heading in the direction of science unleavened by art.

What's the result of insisting that doctors treat patients instead of people? In a 2016 survey of more than 17,000 physicians, *72 percent* said that external factors like third-party authorizations (getting approvals for surgeries and medications and more from insurers and others), treatment protocols, and electronic health record (EHR) design had a substantial *adverse* effect on patient care.[20] (EHR systems are designed to help gather data rather than treat patients, and are a major factor affecting physician morale today, which I'll explore in chapter 6.)

A patient can't be reduced to an algorithm, a step-by-step procedure for solving a problem—where X is one lab result, Y is another, and everything is raised to the power of her age. Patients are unique human beings with a host of factors influencing their health, lifestyle decisions, and the type of treatment plans that will be successful for them. Only a patient's doctor or a medical practice team can understand the full scope of how to give the best care. We need to resist the trend toward treating people and paying doctors based on data and protocols far removed from the reality of a patient's life and their doctor's artful know-how.

I was right, by the way, about those hot red sneakers. They made the perfect gift, and Mike has worn them often over the past nine years. He's loyal to them, because he can feel the care and respect that went into the design of every stitch. And in medicine, we'd all like to see more engaged, loyal patients who get the regular care they need—because when that happens, people can avoid many of the devastating health events everybody worries about.

We need to stop focusing on science and data at all costs. Instead we should be working toward the balance between art and science that will free doctors and medical practice teams to give patients the quality personal care that will engage them most and lead us all, one by one, to become a happier, healthier nation.

The Passion, Power, and Pitfalls of Evidence

On May 7, 2014, a beautiful spring day, thousands of fathers around the country attended the wedding of one of their children. My dad was one of them, but for my brother—the groom—and for our whole family, it was a joyful surprise that Dad was able to be there.

Two days before, as on many other Fridays, my dad was playing cards with the other *alte kakers* at the Jewish Community Center when he noticed that his cards were drooping down toward the table. His left hand was not supporting them. When he tried to raise them, his left arm wouldn't respond, and when he tried to lift his leg, he could barely do so.

Most people in that situation would have called an ambulance or asked a fellow card player for a ride to the hospital. What did Dad do? He got up from the table and dragged his useless arm and almost useless leg out to his car and then *drove himself* ten blocks to the hospital, where he stumbled into the emergency room. (My dad might have invented the concept of DIY the day he was born.) From there, though, the decision-making got a lot better.

Here's a great thing about modern medicine: We know most strokes are caused by a clot that blocks blood flow to the brain. If we can identify a stroke and give the patient tissue plasminogen activator (TPA) to bust up the clot within sixty minutes, the chance of brain damage is dramatically reduced. In medical jargon, it's called door-to-needle, or DTN, time, and from 2003 to 2009 the Target: Stroke national quality improvement initiative worked to help hospitals get their DTN times under sixty minutes. They started with data. What had hospitals done to reduce the time and how had it improved patient outcomes? And then using that data, they created a simple list of strategies and tools to help others achieve similar results.[21] (I've made it sound rather straightforward here, but like any major treatment improvement initiative, it was complex, entailed a lot of education and persuasion, required hospitals to make some significant changes involving more than just their ER departments, and took years to generate real change.)

My father benefited from that work. As soon as he got to the ER, the people there had a plan—a protocol—for how to respond. The nurse on duty saw the paralysis on his left side and immediately called a stroke alert. Within five minutes, he was in a bed with an IV in his arm and an ER physician at his side. He had an initial CT scan, which was read by an on-call neurologist two cities away via telemedicine; that neurologist diagnosed his stroke. My dad was then, per stroke protocol, given the TPA medication. Unfortunately, during his infusion, he developed a headache. They whisked him down for a CT scan to determine if the TPA had caused a bleed in his brain. The neurologist forty miles away read the new scan and gave the good news—it hadn't.

All of this had happened by the time I arrived at the hospital about forty-five minutes after my dad. When I saw him in the bed with the side of his face sagging and his arm limp, I immediately thought of my grandfather, who'd had the same type of stroke when I was ten. Back then, Grandpa spent about ten days in the hospital and a few weeks more in a nursing home before he died a horrible death, due to pneumonia, locked in a lifeless body.

Naturally, my fears grew. It didn't matter that I knew the statistics for stroke victims had improved. This was my *dad*. And no one could really know exactly when his stroke had begun. What if he hadn't arrived at the hospital soon enough? What if we were in for a long-haul recovery, or even something much worse? As I tried to reassure my father, I began preparing myself for whatever might come next.

I'm happy to say that my dad was discharged thirty hours later. The following day, my brother got married. My father attended the wedding, weak on his left side, but alive. Because of modern medicine, Dad was able to offer a somewhat lopsided two-armed bear hug to my brother and his new wife, and enjoy being in the family circle for our celebration of life. The photos from the wedding have extra-special meaning to my brother and I, knowing full well the radically different memories those same photos might have evoked.

Evidence-based medicine—an approach to medical care designed to optimize decision-making by emphasizing the use of evidence from well-designed and well-conducted research—saved my dad, just as it has dramatically improved outcomes for people like him and for people who have heart attacks, severe asthma attacks, complicated pregnancies, and on and on. When it comes to fast, lifesaving treatments for medical emergencies, evidence-based medicine is the gold-medal, stand-up-and-take-a-bow winner. Doctors want a clear path to the absolute best chance of saving a patient's life—whether it's a needle in an arm, a balloon in a closed artery, or a special mask over the nose and mouth that can deliver lifesaving meds instantly. Naturally, when patients are in dire situations, we expect our doctors to rely on the evidence and use helpful data to convert our disease or injury into an entry in the happy-outcome column.

Physicians spend at least eight years studying and another three or more years in training to learn the evidence, *the science*, that will help us make split-second decisions like those made for my dad. Over and over again, we ask: What treatment works best and why? What are the signs of stroke? Of a heart attack? Of specific types of seizures? What do we do first? How do we adjust if the person is twelve? Or eighty-two? We become doctors because we want to learn the answers to these questions—and we have the answers for so many because of thousands of years spent gathering and studying the evidence.

Of course, early on in the history of medicine, the evidence was scarce and understanding of it was ... well, limited. When a woman married in ancient Greece and had trouble conceiving a child, physicians believed her womb—a separate living being with a desire to bear children—had gone a-wandering to some other part of her body. To cure wandering womb, the woman was given foul scents to sniff. Supposedly this would cause the womb to be repelled from its new location and encourage it to return to its rightful spot. And if she hoped to avoid wandering womb altogether, ancient physicians prescribed early marriage, frequent pregnancy, and consistent sex. It's unclear who first came up with that approach, but it was definitely a man.

During the Renaissance and continuing into the twentieth century, physicians used mercury—one of the few elements they could identify—to treat many diseases, especially syphilis. It took quite a while to understand that people might be dying of mercury poisoning rather than syphilis. It did, however, give rise to one of the great phrases of homespun wisdom in medical history: "One night with Venus, a lifetime with Mercury." (Which also definitely came from a dude.)

And of course there's bloodletting, which for millennia was the so-called cure for just about anything, and the standard way to remove "bad blood." (Historians argue that George Washington died due to repeated and excessive bloodletting, totaling more than 80 ounces or 40 percent of his total blood volume, during the last days of his life.) In fact, over the centuries, thousands of odd or repulsive treatments arose for maladies from "bad humors" to "diseased ethers" to the Black Death.

And yet year by year, physician after physician explored, experimented, and studied—each contributing to the progress of modern medical science in his or her own way. According to renowned Egyptologist James Henry Breasted, the first textbook on using a diagnostic approach for spotting and treating disease was written more than 4,600 years ago in Egypt by Imhotep, who many consider to be one of the very first physicians. About 2,000 years ago, the Greek physician Galen published over 500 papers on anatomy, physiology, and more. In 1628, William Harvey published the first comprehensive book on the heart, describing how it pumps blood through the body. Louis Pasteur's work in the 1860s helped physicians everywhere better understand microorganisms, germs, and disease, and spawned a century of vaccine development that altered the future of medicine.

In the last fifty years, the advances have come almost too fast to count, and results keep getting better. Thanks to the work of leaders in the profession, between 1980 and 2000, the rate of coronary heart disease fell by half, saving roughly 341,000 lives *in the year 2000 alone*. Close to half of all those saved lives was a result of better evidence-based therapies.[22] Year after year, physicians and researchers have been advancing the evidence to save the lives of millions, my father among them.

We used to treat heart attacks by sawing through the breastbone to do open-heart surgery, and repairing a torn ligament meant large cuts, obvious scars, and long recovery times. Anesthesia carried big risks all by itself. Now, there is a new wave of drugs making anesthesia safer and better. Most surgeries can be performed laparoscopically—only tiny incisions are needed. Magnetic resonance imaging (MRI) and computed tomography (CT) scans give detailed images of what's going on inside the body. New drugs for the treatment of chronic diseases have fewer side effects.

All this should be great news for doctors and patients—and it is. There's a but, though—one that makes the standard hospital gown look like a flattering outfit by comparison. This tradition of science that doctors are so happy to be part of has advanced at such a wild pace for the last fifty or sixty years, it has become overwhelming. And that is the challenge of modern evidence-based medicine. Recently I read an earnest, sweetly naive piece in defense of evidence-based medicine in its purest form. The author defined it like this: A physician creates a list of search terms based on his patient's condition, inserts them into PubMed or other research database, refines the results "to those articles that are current and deemed of sufficient quality," and then uses the evidence discovered, "applying it to the patient's idiosyncrasies including circumstances, preferences and values."[23] For some reason, I pictured the author wearing a Sherlock Holmes–vintage deerstalker hat as I read this.

Unfortunately, choosing a treatment path often isn't quite so elementary.

Not long ago, one physician wrote, "Medicine is complicated. Sometimes things that seem like they would work just don't pan out."[24] Another said: "We must all understand that science is rarely settled; rather science is always evolving."[25] And what we are all finding is that the standard of "sufficient quality" is hard to define. In fact, it can be downright elusive.

In 1961, Ancel Keys was well known in America, which is a bit unusual for a biochemist. He was on the cover of *Time*, he testified before Congress, and he was quite influential in shaping the diets of Americans for the next sixty years. In 2002, an article in *The Washington Post* declared, "It is difficult to overestimate the importance of Keys's three observations."[26] Keys did foundational research into the relationship between diet and health. A diet high in saturated fats, he told the nation, contributed to bloodstream cholesterol, that selfsame bloodstream cholesterol determined the risk of heart disease, and the people of America were in danger because of our diet.

With a colleague at the University of Minnesota, Ivan Frantz Jr., he conducted one of the largest controlled trials of dietary fat and heart disease, called the Minnesota Coronary Experiment. They found that replacing saturated fats from dairy, eggs, and meat with unsaturated fats from vegetable oils (corn oil) effectively reduced cholesterol. Their reports fed the growth of the war on fat, and in the 1970s, the federal dietary recommendation to replace saturated fats with vegetable oils was codified and is still in place today.

Unfortunately, that may have been a serious mistake.

Several years ago, a medical investigator with the National Institutes of Health named Christopher Ramsden contacted Frantz's son in search of the original records from the study,[27] which were eventually found in the basement of the family home. Ramsden was already looking into other similar studies, and the findings were not what the experts thought. Keys and Frantz tracked mortality (aka whether people live or die) in the study, which oddly did not improve in the trial group. They decided it must be that the experi-

49

ment just wasn't long enough and the trial group not young enough to reveal positive effects.

But when Ramsden and his colleagues finished their analysis of the full data, what they found was that the risk of death actually went up sharply the more cholesterol levels fell, especially in older people. In 2016, they published their findings in the *BMJ*, and started a maelstrom of reexamining what we think we know about saturated fat, cholesterol, diet, and heart disease.[28] Experts are taking sides. People are questioning whether medications to bring down cholesterol are the right choice at all. After all, what—aside from the certainty that the *Simpsons* is on TV every Sunday night— is more ingrained in the American consciousness than the fact that high cholesterol is bad?

Ramsden wasn't the first person to raise a red flag. As far back as the 1990s, others had questioned the standard wisdom, although without all the "evidence" in hand. And even more doctors probably had personal experiences that defied the party line. But if they had decided to voice concerns or opinions, they might have been accused of resisting science. In hindsight, we scoff at the doctors who thought that Louis Pasteur was a nut job, just as we roll our eyes when we think of how few challenged the notion that frontal lobotomies were a legitimate treatment for intellectual disabilities. Yet skepticism may be an important check in our evidence-based world where there's such an emphasis on "new, more, faster."

Of course, healthy skepticism is not a good excuse when sound evidence is simply ignored—and sometimes that happens, too. Not long ago, insurance companies decided they would stop offering coverage for a certain knee surgery. Multiple studies had shown that there was no benefit from it; patients did just as well without any surgical intervention for that particular condition. But doctors wouldn't stop doing the surgery—until the payers made them stop.

In 1997, just twenty years ago, the author of a *Health Affairs* article wrote, "The majority of medical practices are derived not from scientific studies but from 'medical folklore,' with word-of-mouth and a practitioner's past experience determining treatment patterns."[29] He wasn't a doctor, and most doctors at the time would not have agreed, yet what he wrote captures this idea that doctors have to be held accountable to the science. The truth is, most hold *themselves* accountable to the science, doing their best to practice evidence-based medicine. *But we can abide by the science of the day and still get it wrong.*

One day just after Halloween, early in my career, "Thomas" was brought in to the pediatric emergency room (ER). I was moonlighting there in addition to my daytime pediatric practice, and it just so happened that eight-year-old Thomas was a boy I had seen several times at the office.

Thomas wasn't feeling well, and his mom was very concerned because he had no interest whatsoever in his Halloween candy. Looking at him, I started getting a bad feeling in the pit of my stomach. This kid was normally bouncy to the point that he couldn't keep still for more than thirty seconds, yet now he was pale and listless. His mom thought he might have the flu, but she wanted to be sure.

I gently examined the child, who had a temperature of about 100. He flinched when I touched his abdomen. Without other symptoms, the data was ambiguous, because it could fit with a stomach virus or constipation or several other things. Still, my physician intuition was telling me that Thomas had appendicitis.

I asked the on-call surgeon to come in right away, but the surgeon wanted more data to support my diagnosis before he would consent to interrupt his evening. I felt more and more concerned about Thomas, who lay curled up on a hospital bed, his eyes pleading with me to help him. His mom sang to distract him while I drew blood and sent it to the lab. But the results were inconclusive, and the surgeon demanded more data—an abdominal CT scan this time. The scan was also inconclusive. The surgeon still didn't believe this was a bona fide case. Thomas's symptoms were not specific indications of appendicitis.

I had to get someone to listen. "Look, I get it. There is nothing definitive," I said, but then I dropped the gauntlet: "But I know it's an appy, and if you won't come in, I'll get another surgeon." He reluctantly agreed to evaluate the child himself. Minutes after he arrived, he ordered an operating room to be prepared. Soon Thomas was in surgery and his inflamed appendix, near bursting, was removed.

A doctor's instinct to balance the science with the art of medicine to help heal individual patients should not be ignored—because if we choose science or evidence over art consistently, we'll likely get it wrong.

The New Divinity of Data

Meagan was a list maker. A busy mother of two with a master's degree in health administration who was responsible for the hectic office of an orthopedic surgeon, she relied on lists as her bulwark against chaos. When she began feeling sick one spring day, she made an appointment to see her doctor, an internist. True to her habit, she made a list before going in so she could clearly convey her symptoms to her busy doctor.

She had thought she had a yeast infection less than a week before, and treated it with the typical drugstore remedy. But the symptoms hadn't entirely cleared up. Her tissues were still irritated, her urine was dark, and she'd felt a surge of pain in her lower back on both sides, along with getting chills. That was when she knew it was time to see a doctor. The last item on the list in her trusty, carry-everywhere Day Planner: "Had vag strep once before. Am I contagious?"

At her appointment, her internist did a quick exam and told her that he believed she was coming down with the flu. It was still flu season, after all, so it was a likely diagnosis. He also did a pelvic exam and told her that the red rash was yeast hanging on. He prescribed two meds—one for the yeast and one to curb the flu virus—and then sent her home to rest up and drink plenty of fluids.

If you're trained in medicine, you might already realize how wrong the doctor was. Meagan thought he might be wrong, too, because her concern was the back pain, she later told her husband, which didn't fit entirely into either diagnosis. But she followed the advice she'd been given. A few days later, a Sunday, she called the office and spoke to the doctor on call, and the next day she came back in. She needed a wheelchair to get from the car to the office. Her blood pressure was so low, they couldn't detect it. They called an ambulance and she was rushed to the nearest hospital and admitted into intensive care. Sadly, the next day she died—of toxic-shock syndrome from a rampant group A strep infection that had started in her vagina and then spread to her internal organs. She was just forty-six years old.

Patrick Malone, the attorney and patient safety advocate who represented her family in their malpractice suit against the doctor, shared her story in *The Life You Save*, a book on the steps you can take to get the best health care.[30] Sadly, Meagan's story is not an anomaly at its base. Incorrect or missed diagnoses are common in our health-care system, so common that some experts have predicted that they will happen at least once to every person in America. In 2014, the journal *BMJ Quality & Safety* published the results of a study that estimates the number of people who are misdiagnosed each year at about *12 million*.[31]

Why? Certainly, ignored science and protocols play a role. In Meagan's case, the internist didn't do a vaginal culture and didn't draw blood. In other words, relevant scientific evidence wasn't gathered, a tragically sloppy mistake. But if the internist had relied on the art of medicine and listened to what the patient had to say, it might have encouraged better science. His patient described her symptoms and asked whether she might have vaginal strep; Meagan essentially told him exactly what was wrong with her—and he didn't listen. In fact, though he typed notes into the electronic health record, he didn't record most of the symptoms Meagan had on her list. Malone suggests that, given Meagan's habits and communication style, it was unlikely she made a list and then didn't mention what was on it. "Either he hadn't heard what she said," Malone wrote, "or he hadn't asked her the thorough questions, body system by body system, that would have teased out her full story."

Abraham Verghese is a physician, Stanford professor, and award-winning writer. "The high-tech transformation of medical care has resulted in diminishing direct patient-physician interaction," he and his colleagues wrote when they published the results of a survey they'd conducted.[32] In their survey, doctors asked their colleagues to recount stories of conditions, illnesses, wounds and more that were missed during a physical examination. From the stories they received, the team generated a list of 206, from broken legs and arms and hernias, to large masses in the abdomen and signs of heart attack or heart disease, to appendicitis and pregnancies—even in one woman who was in labor! Some items in the list are incredibly sad: "Missed pregnancy with twins before hysterectomy," "Missed bruising signs of abuse in child," "Missed breast cancer." Others are ruefully ridiculous: "Missed previous appendectomy scar and made diagnosis of appendicitis" and "Missed watch battery in umbilicus [belly button] in child."

At Stanford Medical School, Verghese leads the Stanford Medicine 25, a program focused on training interns and residents in the twenty-five most crucial bedside exam skills. Take a moment to ponder that. One of the best medical schools in the country has had to launch a special program to focus attention on what was once—not long ago in the history of medicine—the *only* method of diagnosing a patient. More important, it has always, always been essential to the art of *treating* a patient—as a human being who needs healing. Is there better proof that science, data, and technology are overstepping and overshadowing the art of medicine?

Today many doctors are being taught that treating a patient begins and ends with data—what we learn from a medical record and what we put into it. They are being encouraged to prioritize the data over the patient's story. A long-time doctor I know who has conducted hospital rounds with medical students forever now refers to them as the "circles of tablets," since every student carries and consults information on their tablet computer before ever looking at the patient. They attend to the EHR (the holy repository) more than they attend to the tale that the patient and the patient's physical body have to tell. They do this despite the proof that doctors who have completely avoided malpractice suits tend to spend more time with their patients and focus on the artful work of drawing out their patients' views of what's happening.[33] They do this in large part because of demands for more and more data, and because they are told to trust the data more than the patient.

Since the advent of Big Data and recent technological innovations, the care and connection doctors want to provide seem to be pushed to the background—along with the big picture of the patient. Riding shotgun are the thousands upon thousands of different guidelines, protocols, and checklists from societies, hospitals, health plans, and the Centers for Medicare and Medicaid Services (CMS) regulations. All of these end up governing a whopping percentage of the decisions made by doctors—all because we are able to gather and process the numbers from millions of patient encounters to create averages that inform, or even dictate, that decision-making.

When doctors say "evidence-based medicine," there's often an eye-roll, and that's because "evidence-based" has come to represent a rather infuriating basket of requirements: more treatment protocols, ever more data to back up those protocols, and a high volume of tasks (like requesting preauthorization) to prove that those protocols are being followed. Just imagine a teacher that has to check with outside experts every fifteen minutes before teaching a lesson, or a ballerina having a teacher yell out every specific movement before completing it. Everywhere doctors turn today, they bump up against another request for data to be entered into the health record, another protocol-based alert or checklist, and more insistence that they attend to it rather than the patient. It's as if a baseball catcher were required to keep a detailed record

55

of every single pitch he caught—the location of it, how he caught it, how fast it was traveling, whether it was the pitch he called for or not, and whether it got hit—after every single batter, keeping the pitcher and everybody else waiting. These daily, often hourly, requirements have been on the rise since the 1980s with the rise of managed care, the HMO, and federal regulation—about the same time, incidentally, that other industries were beginning to talk about customization for customers.

Is anyone surprised that in a recent survey, doctors revealed that the least satisfying aspects of the job are regulatory or paperwork burdens and the erosion of clinical autonomy?[34] It is undoubtedly frustrating to deal with the demands to collect data and efforts by payers and regulators to dictate how doctors should practice based on that data. Never mind that patient-centered care happens at the personal level, taking into account the individual's unique health factors, life situation, job, relationships, personal choices and opinions, and personality.

There is an important time and place for data and protocols in medicine. That time is not always, and that place is not everywhere.

If You Can't, We Will

I attend a *lot* of health-care conferences. For the last few years, I've gone to fifteen or twenty a year. It comes with the job. My one regret is that in the last couple of years I haven't been able to attend the South by Southwest (or SXSW) interactive conference in Austin, Texas, which includes a health and medtech track in its five days of all things tech-related. You might be more familiar with SXSW's roots as a music, interactive technology, and film conference, but in America today, if you're talking about the market for technological innovation, you have to talk about health care—because that's where the money is.

Here's the setup at SXSW: People vote for the sessions they want the producers to include based on a list of proposed panel discussions. When you're competing for votes and for audience members, you have to be provocative in your choice of session title. The blue-ribbon title on the roster for 2016, at least in my book, was "Pimp My Brain: A Crash Course in DIY Brainhacking"—a ghastly idea, but I would probably have attended, that is, as long as it didn't conflict with "Giving the Tricorder Life Fifty Years After Star Trek."

In the last three years, if you read through the list of medtech session titles, you might have picked up on a theme—the person-alization and customization that people are beginning to expect in health care, apparently including the ability to do bizarre things to their own brains in the comfort of their living rooms. Sessions like "iDiet, iDid-It! Losing Weight with Wearables," "Know Thyself: Introspective Personal Data Mining," "Home, Sweet Home: The Health Hub of the Future," "Imagining the Future of Personalized Medicine," "It's Like Uber for Healthcare," "Wearables: The Powder Keg for a Health Revolution," and "The Return of Psychedelic Re-search in America." (I'm just assuming that last one is an idea being pushed by patients—most likely, aging Baby Boom hippy patients who think of Wavy Gravy as more than a Ben & Jerry's flavor.)

Tech innovators are stepping in to seize an opportunity. Patients who feel they're getting by-the-numbers health care are turning to technology to design their own health experiences and achieve their own health goals. On the surface, it sounds wonderful, but I doubt people really want their health care to come from robots, no matter how good the tricorders—handheld medical devices that read vital signs in seconds—are. And frankly the tricorders, at least in the form of health apps, are not so good yet. One study published in the journal *BMJ* found that diagnosis apps or symptom check-ers put the right answer at the top of the list of possible condi-tions only about 34 percent of the time, and put it in the top twenty only 58 percent of the time.[35] Honestly, if Dr. McCoy's tricorder was correct only 34 percent of the time when diagnosing Captain Kirk, the good doctor wouldn't be the only one who's always yell-ing, "Dammit!" Patients themselves don't do much better using online information. In one study, older people determined the right cause of their symptoms based on online information less than half the time.[36]

One day my mom called me out of the blue. "Halee," she said, "I need to tell you where the safe is and the combination so you can have my jewelry when I'm gone."

I asked her why she was bringing this up *now*. "Well, I've been having pain and tingling in my hands, and I looked this symptom up on WebMD. I have ALS." (If you haven't diagnosed yourself with ALS, also known as Lou Gehrig's Disease, you may not know that it is a disease of the nervous system that weakens muscles, eventually causing paralysis. It is the disease that afflicts Stephen Hawking.)

Honestly, this wasn't the first conversation I'd had like this with my mom, but it was definitely one of the more unexpected self-diagnoses she'd come up with. (And if you're wondering whether my mother used to bundle me up in so many layers before I could play in the snow that she practically made me a portable heater, the answer is yes.)

I said, "Really?"

"Yes, I looked through all the symptoms and it matches." She then listed the symptoms of general fatigue, blurry vision, muscle tiredness, and pain and tingling in her hands.

"Fascinating, Mom."

"Promise me you'll take care of your dad and your brothers?" Her voice caught in her throat; she was trying not to cry.

"Nope."

"Why not?"

"Mom, you don't have ALS."

"Yes I do. I looked it up on WebMD and then I googled the symptoms to make sure."

"Uh-huh."

"Don't 'uh-huh' me, Halee. This is serious. I'm going to die a horrible death soon."

"No, Mom. You aren't. You are going to live for a really long time, and I'm afraid to tell you, you'll be pretty healthy doing it— you've got great genetics. By the way, thank you for that gift."

"But I'm telling you, my vision is blurry and my hands are tingling and—"

"Mom, how much have you been working?" (My mom's an accountant, and it was tax season.)

"Oh, I don't know—maybe twelve- or fourteen-hour days."

"On a computer?" I prompted.

"Yes."

"Sitting the whole time?" I pursued.

"Yes."

"So you don't think your blurry vision and your tingling hands have anything to do with overuse injuries?"

"No."

"Huh. Have you talked to Bill [her doctor] about your diagnosis?" I asked.

"Not yet."

"Why don't you call him and tell him your diagnosis and mention that I think you should get a B-12 shot," I said.

"Why B-12?"

"Well, besides overuse being a cause of your issues, Grandma— your mother—has a B-12 deficiency that can give you tingling ... so you may, too. She gets a B-12 shot every month."

"She does?"

"Yep."

"Oh."

"Uh-huh."

James Madara, current head of the American Medical Association, has called health apps and tech products "the digital snake oil of the early twenty-first century."[37] His point? Technology alone will not deliver health results. A study published in the fall of 2016 found that devices like the Fitbit or Jawbone are not much better than buying a gym membership. They have an immediate effect on people's fitness levels, but most users slip back into their old habits within six months.[38]

In his 2015 book *The Patient Will See You Now*, Eric Topol tells readers the stories of three different plane rides during which a passenger was sick and he was asked to step in as a doctor. Each time, digital technology on his smartphone allowed him to diagnose a heart-related problem. He concluded, "Although the flight crew had asked if there were doctors on board, all that was needed were the tools to collect the data."[39] And yet in each situation, he interpreted the data *based on his decades of experience as a cardiologist.* He then made a judgment call about whether the plane needed to make an emergency landing or not. So tools to collect data were *not* all that was needed. Now Topol assumes that the data could be sent to somebody on the ground who could interpret it, but I wonder how well that would work. First, if sick people use the tool and mistakenly believed they have understood the information completely, maybe they won't try to communicate with a health professional. And even if they did, what might be missed in a long-distance data-based assessment? A lot, I think. And from Topol's own experiences with his knee replacement, which I shared in the last chapter, we know how he feels about by-the-protocol care.

All that said, health tech has amazing potential to change the ability of patients and physicians to customize and personalize experiences—to make data gathering easier and less time-consuming, allowing more room for the art of medicine. In chapter 8, I'll tell you a bit about how one company is forging the way forward by giving patients access to their electronic health records. Patients are then given tools to help them track and report vitals and other results that empower them and their care team to manage their chronic conditions. This patient-centric approach is rare, though. And the current technology available to people is not the answer, it's just a set of tools.

If we want patients to be healthier, it's going to take more than 10,000 steps a day or another way to store and track their personal data. Health-care providers must engage them in the decisions made, and that will take more than sending lab results or spouting protocols. That will take time, freedom, and flexibility.

When it comes to scientific information, I believe that the smartest physicians are those just out of medical school. Science is every med student's forte because students are expected to absorb so much knowledge and recite it at any moment, especially during their internship and then residency, when they're learning to apply it to real human bodies. And eventually they have to pass their licensing and board exams.

Now imagine someone you love is ill. You have a choice between two physicians. One has been practicing for nine months, is fresh out of training, and carries massive amounts of scientific knowledge around in his head. The other has been practicing for nine years, and in addition to a knowledge of medicine has developed intuitive skills born of experience with living patients. Which doctor would you choose?

I'll tell you the choice my husband, Mike, and I made when he was diagnosed with kidney cancer less than a month after I gave him his fantastic red sneakers. First, though, let me tell you what we as doctors didn't do. We didn't check the current protocols for treatment. We didn't go to PubMed and look up the recent research. We didn't even go online and google his diagnosis—in fact, we especially did not do that. We were in crisis, we were vulnerable, and we put our faith, our hope, and Mike's life in his experienced physician's hands—a physician we knew we could trust to treat Mike as a whole, human being, not just a collection of data points. I'm grateful for that decision every day of our lives. I believe her artful practice of medicine, guided by her extensive experience with the best science, is what saved Mike.

To feel good about our own experiences in health care always needs something more than the successful completion of a procedure or a correct prescription. Practicing the art of medicine does not detract from the science, does not weaken it. The art enhances the science, making it more likely to be effective, and more engaging for the human beings who show up in the exam room.

"I will remember that there is art to medicine as well as science, and that warmth, sympathy, and understanding may outweigh the surgeon's knife or the chemist's drug."

This line from a modern version of the Hippocratic oath should guide the industry just as it is designed to guide the individual doctor.

CHAPTER 4

The Lever to Move Medicine

Business is the driver of change in health care,
for better or for worse.

EVERY SELF-RESPECTING fan of television in the 1990s should be able to tell you exactly where they were on the night of November 9, 1995. Here's a hint for the TV nerds out there: It was a Thursday.

This was the night that Dr. Doug Ross—rakish bad boy and womanizer who habitually came to work hung over and was about to be fired from his job—morphed into Dr. Doug Ross, reluctant hero, when he rescues a young boy stuck behind a locked grate in a metal storm tunnel as the waters from a torrential downpour rise around them.

And, oh yeah, he did it while wearing a tuxedo.

Mike and I were medical residents living in a small rented apartment in Phoenix, Arizona, at the time, and we'll never forget watching that episode from the second season of *ER*. Very few actors have ever had a money shot quite like the one that George Clooney's Ross had after he and the boy are propelled out of the tunnel and into a lake. Ross has to find the kid underwater and dives three times, staying under just long enough to make the tension unbearable. He finally breaks through the water with the boy in his arms. As the storm pelts their faces, a spotlight from a TV helicopter hovering above shines down on them. Bathed in light, the doctor slowly raises the boy Christ-like to the skies above, then nearly sinks below the waves getting the kid to shore because the director had hired a young actor who weighed nearly as much as Clooney. Dr. Ross eventually saves the boy and becomes a star.

"Hell and High Water" is the episode that launched Clooney into the stratosphere. It was riveting and iconic and insanely over the top. For years afterward, when friends asked me to name my favorite episodes from medical dramas (as my geeky friends are wont to do), I never included it—because to me, it seemed more like an action-adventure than something that would actually happen between a medical professional and a patient.

That is, until I heard the story of "Gloria Brown"[40] and Hurricane Sandy—which is also one of my favorite stories about the business of medicine.[41]

Twelve weeks before Sandy became the largest Atlantic hurricane on record, Gloria was feeling ill and visited her doctor. After a series of tests, it was confirmed that she had hepatitis C. The more she heard about it from her doctor, the more scared she became.

Hepatitis C, she learned, is a disease that attacks the liver and damages it over time. Afflicting four million Americans and more than 150 million people worldwide, it is a disease that affects roughly five times as many people around the globe as the number infected with HIV, the virus that causes AIDS. Like HIV, hep C is also spread through needle sharing, blood transfusions, and sex—her doctor guessed that she had contracted it through a blood transfusion two decades before. When Gloria wondered how that was possible, her doctor explained that hep C works so quietly that it can damage the liver for decades before any symptoms occur. By the time it's found, it's usually too late.

The good news, Gloria was told, was that her condition was likely caught in time. There was one medication in particular that had a good chance of curing her, as long as she didn't miss a single dose. If she did, she could quickly develop a resistance to the drug, making it ineffective and likely resigning her to suffering for the rest of her life. The bad news, though, was that the drug was known to have punishing side effects. If she could endure treatment every day for twelve weeks, she would likely be cured. She decided to try.

The first few weeks went well. But then the side effects hit, and hit hard. As Patrick Thean reveals in his book *Rhythm*, Gloria developed a rash and bleeding hemorrhoids. A fiery itch covered "every square inch" of her body. Mouth sores made it painful for her to eat, and extremely dry skin made her feel like she was on fire. Summoning the strength she needed, she somehow kept going. After six weeks, she received fantastic news: a blood test confirmed that the virus was no longer detected in her body. If she could endure the pain and misery she felt for another six weeks, she would likely be cured.[42] In late October of 2012, she ordered the next batch of her treatment and waited for it to be rush-delivered to her New Jersey home.

Unfortunately, Hurricane Sandy arrived first.

The powerful storm hit land at the Jersey Shore not far from Gloria's house on October 29, battering everything in its path with its sustaining 80 mph winds. By the time it was over, thirty-seven people were dead, nearly 350,000 homes were damaged or destroyed, huge swaths of the state were underwater, and two million households—including Gloria's—were out of power. Meanwhile, Gloria's medication was stuck far away, in a distribution center in another state.

While she grieved for her state, Gloria was despondent about her disease. She knew that if she missed even a single day of treatment, all of the suffering she had endured would have been for naught. She couldn't believe that she would have to start all over, or worse—she might never again be able to receive the treatment she needed to save her life. For Gloria, Hurricane Sandy felt more like a death sentence.[43]

That's when an unlikely champion sprang into action.

BioPlus Specialty Pharmacy doesn't sound much like an action hero. It's hard to imagine it adorned with boots and a cape. Truth be told, it sounds more like something Dr. Evil might cook up to

65

take on Austin Powers or the antagonist in one of the X-Men movies. But BioPlus wasn't just the company that had shipped Gloria's medication to her, it was the one that had invented the therapy in the first place. In fact, for many physicians and patients across America, BioPlus Specialty Pharmacy already had a reputation as miracle workers.

Their genius came in the way they improved the function of intravenous medication, also known as that tube that gets stuck in your vein as medicine gets dripped from an IV bag above you. It's called "drip" for a reason—those drips last for hours. Unfortunately, there are many medications that have to enter the body slowly through a vein. Before companies like BioPlus, you would need to either check in to a hospital or go to an IV infusion facility—which, I can tell you from my own experience, isn't like sitting on your most comfortable chair with your Big Bird slippers propped up on your coffee table at home.

Some years ago, I was involved in saving a dog from being hit by a car. Long story short, I was bitten by the rescued dog and developed a serious hand infection that needed a week of IV antibiotic therapy. My doctor sent me to a hospital infusion center, and soon it was my turn to get a needle shoved in my arm. The meds stung as they dripped and it seemed to take forever and a day before the IV bag was finally empty. That wasn't all, because I still had to come back several times. I felt like I was in purgatory, and I wasn't even sick, aside from the infection.

If I'd had cancer or an immune disorder or hemophilia, my experience would have been much worse—true hell because the treatment time would have taken six to eight hours instead of two, and I would have felt weak when I came in and weaker still when I left.

Enter the magic of BioPlus. For years, they had built their reputation on easing the way for patients whose doctors prescribed specialized medications—patients who needed treatment for uncommon or difficult-to-treat conditions like hep C. Treatments could be expensive and complicated. Too often, patients like Gloria would

66

experience the horrible side effects and stop treatment because of all the other hurdles that came with the pain.

Dr. Stephen C. Vogt, CEO and founder of BioPlus, wanted to do something about that. From his headquarters in Altamonte Springs, Florida, Dr. Vogt and his team reengineered IVs, making them work better, faster—and at home. Which is how BioPlus came to be responsible for shipping a package with medication to Gloria Brown's house in New Jersey, which now sat like a ticking clock in a distribution center a state away.

One of the benefits to being headquartered in Florida is that BioPlus has a lot of experience with hurricanes. From the moment that Hurricane Sandy hit land in New Jersey, the team at BioPlus overseeing Gloria's therapy contacted hospitals and doctors in the area to see if anybody had even a few doses of the medication that they could spare, but nobody did. The team then reached out to local specialty pharmacies to see if anybody had the medication in-store, to effectively hand treatment of Gloria over to them, but again, nobody did. The clock was running down and the team knew it was time for drastic measures.

Here's the BioPlus version of getting tossed out of a storm drain and diving underwater to save a kid in a lake: In the end, they chartered a private jet to fly a refrigerated batch of Gloria's medication to the closest airport accepting flights in New Jersey. Then they found a private courier amid the hurricane devastation, who met the plane as it landed and then drove directly to Gloria, placing the package in her grateful hands—just one hour shy of the scheduled treatment time.

The BioPlus team did all of this without ever contacting their CEO. Why? Because they knew their actions were in keeping with the mission of BioPlus. In his book *Rhythm*, Patrick Thean shared this story as an example of the power of purpose and values to drive growth in successful organizations. Gloria Brown is one of the beneficiaries of that purpose.

It wasn't always this way. A few years ago, BioPlus's growth was slowing and they needed to understand how to do better if they wanted to outpace their competitors. Drugmakers don't allow just any pharmacy to distribute these medications because they are expensive to produce in small quantities and require special handling and storage. Naturally, patients who are prescribed these meds need much more support than the typical pharmacy can provide. Physicians want to know that their patients will receive that support. BioPlus needed to consider how they could continue to make their programs attractive to doctors and pharmaceutical companies. They began by going to the doctors who referred patients to them to ask about their experiences. *Your outcomes are great,* they heard, *but you're hard to do business with.*

The difficulties were many, but BioPlus didn't cause them.

In many ways, they had what I like to call a "Jessica Rabbit problem." In the animated film *Who Framed Roger Rabbit,* Jessica was a voluptuous character who utters the memorable line "I'm not bad. I'm just drawn that way." BioPlus wasn't badly managed or inefficient—but it was subject to the inefficient way the prescription medication industry had been drawn around it. The chief culprit was the 2003 Medicare Prescription Drug, Improvement, and Modernization Act, which requires doctors to use electronic systems to transmit prescriptions to pharmacies. The problem is, those systems are not always compatible between medical practices, pharmacies, and the insurance companies and government programs that pay the bills. The biggest hurdle is that most specialty medications require preauthorization because they are so expensive (from $1,000 to $10,000 per month). "There is not a doctor's office in the country that is built to withstand all the administrative overhead required to successfully navigate the barriers to getting a patient started on a specialty medication," Dr. Elvin Montanez, COO at Bio-Plus, said recently. "Our retail customer's number one need is time saved."[44] In other words, we're talking about mountains of paperwork, multiple gigabits of storage, and hours of phone calls, all of which take time, time, and more time.

They did, however, find a way to fix them.

What did BioPlus do? They set about tackling time.

First, they pledged to knock the timeline for finding out if a patient's health plan would cover the treatment down from two to three days to two hours. With a major investment in staff and technological innovation (building a proprietary prescription system), they did it. This set them apart and allowed them to break into new markets faster. They also developed contracts with more pharmaceutical companies.

Next, they took up authorization denials from insurance companies. It's not uncommon for insurers to deny coverage for these medications. Once coverage is denied, providers must submit an appeal and make an airtight clinical case for why the treatment is necessary, which of course is hugely time-consuming. Last year, BioPlus took that task off the shoulders of medical practices. To do that, they've had to employ a team of clinicians to review patient files and pull together all the right information to convince insurers of the wisdom and necessity of treatment plans. But hallelujah, an amazing 80 percent of their appeals are approved.

BioPlus shares their vision on their website: "The BioPlus Way is to deliver specialty pharmacy solutions that measurably improve adherence to a plan of care, ensure optimal therapeutic outcomes, and lighten the administrative burden of physicians' offices, all while ensuring moral, legal, and ethical conduct."

By fulfilling that vision, BioPlus has grown its revenue by 150 percent every year for the last three years.

All right, let's take a pause while I ask: Does that last detail about revenue make you respect BioPlus less? Does it reduce the value of their work and their commitment, in your eyes, because they're profiting from it? If you had read that sentence at the *beginning* of this chapter, before reading about Gloria Brown, would it have put you in a different frame of mind about the company?

Well, I'm about to share something so controversial in my profession that I may well get my doctor card revoked: I'm glad that

BioPlus is profitable. In fact, I'm one of the people who believes we're lucky that the business of medicine is booming. If BioPlus, with all their helpful ways and their belief in patient care, had to struggle to keep their doors open, I'd be even more worried about the future of health care. Instead, their profits give me hope.

I call BioPlus a unicorn because they're a rare animal in the forest of health care—one that embodies the balance of art, *business, and science* in medicine. This balance supports the best outcomes. So if companies like BioPlus can show the whole industry that balance can happen *while also creating a sustainable company*, they might just lead the way into a much better future. Along the way, they might also make it easier for a majority of my physician peers to speak the phrase "the business of medicine" without spitting out their coffee in the process.

As Archimedes once said, "Give me a place to stand, and with a lever I will move the whole world." (Not to be confused with Margaret Thatcher, who said, "I shan't be pulling the levers there, but I shall be a very good backseat driver." That's not what we want.) Standing within the circle of the art and science of medicine, I see the business of medicine as the lever for the outcomes we hope for in health care today. It's the link to the marketplace that drives innovation and medical discovery. It creates access to health care so that physicians can practice the art of medicine with more patients who desperately need it. With this lever, the whole world of health care can be changed for the better for everyone.

First, though, we have to recognize the conflict many people involved in delivering health care feel when it comes to achieving the efficiency and profitability business requires to be sustainable with the art or the human care required to make the practice of medicine effective. Finding balance that resolves that conflict, like BioPlus did and like others have done, requires that those in the business of medicine adopt a vision for the powerful positive force the business of medicine can play in our health-care future.

The Lever Arm

One of the great and slightly intimidating things about living in Denver is how many super-healthy people you meet on a daily basis.

You might have a conversation in the morning with a friend who ran a half marathon over the weekend, chat with a coworker in the afternoon who is training for a triathlon, and exchange pleasantries in the evening with a plucky neighbor who took advantage of her day off to ride her bike fifty miles over the mountains while still getting in a little skiing before it got dark. What it means for the rest of us is that we have to be really selective whom we talk with about that Ben & Jerry's Cherry Garcia we may or may not have eaten on Saturday night while watching *The Shawshank Redemption*.

But even by Colorado standards, Chau Smith is an inspiration. In early 2017, there was a CNN story about the Missourian that said she wasn't content to run four marathons in five weeks, or ten marathons a year. Instead, she challenged herself and successfully ran seven marathons on seven continents in seven days, which is known as the Triple 7 Quest. To prepare for it, she ran up to 130 miles each week for four months. A year earlier, she ran a marathon in Tanzania and, not quite tired enough, climbed Kilimanjaro the next day.

There's one other thing I forgot to mention: Chau Smith is seventy years old.

What's maybe most remarkable of all is that while Smith's story is extreme, versions of it are being repeated by older Americans across the country, who are experiencing a quality of life in later years that is a departure from what came before. It's not for nothing that Jo Ann Jenkins, the CEO of AARP, wrote a book called *Disrupt Aging*, the central thesis of which is that we need to begin rethinking institutions and long-held norms because people are living much longer than before. Indeed, a session at the 2017 World Economic Forum in Davos was dedicated to the topic "Preparing for the 100-Year Life." The purpose was to address the reality that by the year 2050, there will be more people over the age of sixty than under the age of fifteen for the first time in history.

These things have not happened by accident. They are the result of a new generation who has therapies, treatments, and medications to extend life in ways their parents and grandparents never had. All of it came courtesy of the innovators, funders, inventors, and payers at the heart of our health-care industry. The business of medicine will only get bigger as our population ages and as more people develop chronic disease, seek more treatments, and take more meds. Retirees today will most likely live longer than their parents, manage more disease than their parents, and utilize breakthroughs in treatments not available to their parents. And all of that must be supported by the business of medicine.

Why, then, does the phrase "business of medicine" raise visions of a good-versus-evil battle for the soul of patient-centered health care? I can give you a list of more than two dozen doctors I know who think discussing money is vulgar. That's great, I usually say to them, but everyone else is talking about it, so maybe you should be, too.

If we get real about it, isn't good business essential to the successful delivery of care in our country? Without good business, the daily practice of medicine would need its own trip to an infusion center. Good business for medical practices facilitates good health. Backed by good business, the art of medicine can flourish, helping more patients and serving healthier communities. Good business means there's money available to fund research into new tests, technology, treatments, and cures. Because you know all those double-blind studies and clinical trials aren't cheap. Without funding, they simply wouldn't get done. When good business pays for care, patients get more access to medical services than at any other time in history.

That's all great. Do you feel the "but" that's on its way?

Well, good business also means efficient use of resources—

which is code for cutting costs and reducing waste. And for the last fifty-plus years, the demands of the business of medicine have interfered with the art of medicine more and more. Because "efficiency" brings us back to the issue of time.

Efficiency doesn't recognize that a weeping patient needs time to wipe his tears before he can tell a doctor his symptoms; that a doctor confronted with a mysterious illness needs time to do a more thorough exam, order more tests, and review all the information. Efficiency tends to look down its nose at the time it takes for doctors to build trust with their patients, to reassure them, and to get the full story of what's going on in their lives.

There's that word again: *time*.

If efficiency in medicine gets defined with formulas such as number of billable hours divided by number of patients seen, number of tests performed multiplied by average costs for each test, or number of referrals given compared to national average, where does that leave the art of medicine? When doctors are forced to focus on efficiency for efficiency's sake, they cannot do what they need to do because the time it takes for the art of medicine is eaten up by other tasks and other considerations—such as whether a service will be paid for. I'm not opposed to reducing waste or achieving lower costs, but only if those things are done with the patient's welfare first and foremost—meaning only if the time needed to carry out the art of medicine is factored in. If art is absent, all of the business processes in the world won't achieve the desired results.

This isn't exactly a phenomenon unique to medicine. After all, if the owners of the Pittsburgh Steelers wanted one of their linebackers to play better, they wouldn't prescribe to the coach of the linebackers the exact defensive schemes they wanted the linebacker to study and the drills they wanted him to run, and how the game film should be broken down to help the linebacker learn. Instead, they would provide what the coach needed to do the job, and then rely upon the coach to teach his art to the player based on his judgment, talent, and experience. It's about recognizing the specific

73

roles and responsibilities each member of the team has in achieving the ultimate goals.

Ironically, the art of medicine is essential to achieving those lower costs and the reduced waste. Yes, as we've seen, when physicians have more time to spend with patients rather than dealing with the laundry list of requirements to get reimbursed by most payers, guess what happens? Fewer patients end up coming back a week later for another illness, and fewer patients go undiagnosed, which keeps them out of emergency rooms.

It would be much truer to the values of efficiency if fewer patients would go to the ER (an ER visit is much more expensive, by a multiple of ten-plus, because of the infrastructure hospitals have to maintain—the staff, the equipment, the labs, and of course the liability insurance), and yet the rules established in the name of efficiency have led to more people using the emergency room. Why? Because they don't visit a primary care doctor on a regular basis, someone who would catch a larger health issue before it got bad enough to bring on an emergency.

So where do we go from here?

A Little Tough Love for the Business of Medicine

I travel frequently, and being a social person, I'll strike up conversations with the people I sit next to on a plane. We'll exchange names, professions, and number of kids or pets. If the person next to me is over the age of forty, when they find out I'm a physician, they invariably share with me their version of idyllic health-care days, when their doctors were just like the TV doctors we grew up worshiping, and not the obstacles they have to navigate around now.

I'm not immune to those ideals of yesteryear. I even have my own real-life idol, my pediatrician, Dr. Jules Amer. In a blue coat with his name embroidered on it, his hands smelling like Dove soap, and wearing shoes he'd purchased from my dad many, many, many years earlier, Jules was an ex officio member of more fami-

74

lies than he could count. If you visited his office, you were guaranteed a two-hour wait in the crowded, Lysol-smelling waiting room, which was just fine, since you knew he was going to spend an hour with you. He knew his patients from when they were born, when they had babies (he had been my mom's pediatrician), and when their babies had babies, without the interference of insurers or drug companies or advanced technology.

During the orientation lecture on my first day of medical school, one of the deans asked who in the class had had Dr. Amer as a pediatrician, and 9 out of 125 students raised their hands. The dean wasn't surprised at all. It had been that way for almost twenty-five years. If you're going to choose a role model, you'd better make it a good one, and Dr. Amer remains the very best role model for what the art of medicine has the power to be. Most of us have physician heroes—but what we often forget is the unsung hero of business that underlies all that inspiring art.

Meet someone who benefited greatly from that business. In 2011, Philip Mason began to lose his hair. It's not uncommon for a seventy-year-old retiree to suffer hair loss, but it was the way it happened that seemed weird. His hair wasn't just falling off his head, it was falling from his entire body. Then he began to lose weight, dropping twenty-five pounds in such a short amount of time that he felt nauseated and weak. Soon after came the falls. Blind since birth, Philip already walked with a white cane, but he decided to switch to a walker. The former computer programmer visited his doctor and after a series of tests, heard terrible news: hepatitis C. Because Philip was already suffering from a chronic condition in his kidneys, his prognosis wasn't good: The infection was so advanced that the doctor recommended a transplant. But Philip worried that a transplant—with the long recovery, the lifetime of anti-rejection drugs, and more—would have negative, long-lasting effects on his quality of life.

Philip did have other options, though. One was the therapy Bio-Plus delivered to Gloria in our opening story, which consisted of regular injections of interferon and other drugs for months to boost the immune system, a program that cured up to seven in ten patients. But those injections often came with terrible side effects, as we've already learned.[45] Instead, Philip chose the option also chosen by Keith Richards, Mickey Mantle, and Pamela Anderson: Live with it.

That's what he did until February 2014, when he visited his doctor for a checkup. His doctor asked if he'd like to try a new drug that had just come on the market a few months earlier and showed promising results. It was a simple yellowish pill called sofosbuvir, known better by the brand name Sovaldi. As he later recounted for a story in Vox,[46] Philip was told that all he'd need to do was take the Sovaldi pill along with one other medication once a day for twelve weeks.

Shortly into his treatment, something wonderful happened. Philip's hair started to grow back. He gave up his walker. He no longer felt weak. And three weeks after he finished treatment, another great result: Tests showed that his hepatitis C was completely gone. Of course, by the numbers, this wasn't all that surprising. Since it was approved by the Food and Drug Administration in December 2013, Sovaldi has achieved a staggering cure rate of 90 percent, with very few side effects. In essence, it has turned a difficult-to-treat illness into one that's easy to manage—and cure—in three months.

Developed by a small New Jersey biotechnology firm called Pharmasset and distributed by pharmaceutical giant Gilead Sciences, Sovaldi was invented by a child of Italian immigrants named Michael Sofia. He was drawn to Pharmasset for the reputation it had earned for chemically altering the building blocks of DNA and RNA, known as nucleosides, in ways that snapped the chains of the genetic code, potentially stopping deadly viruses in their tracks.

Problem was, nucleoside drugs hadn't been used for hep C because they couldn't enter liver cells. Sofia's genius was to find a way to create a Harry Potter–like "invisibility cloak" for the drug to get it into the liver. When liver cells attacked the cloak, the drug would activate—trapping it in the liver and preventing it from traveling anywhere else in the body, curing the viral disease without creating side effects.[47] For his historic contribution to medical science, Sofia was awarded the prestigious Lasker Award, often seen as the predictor of a Nobel Prize.

For the right to distribute the lifesaving drug, Gilead paid more than $11 billion.

To put that in context, in 1970, the entire United States spent $75 billion TOTAL on health care—for EVERYTHING.

Thanks in large part to the breakthroughs enabled by organized medical research like the Gileads of the world, since 1970, death rates for heart disease have dropped more than 60 percent and deaths from stroke by more than 70 percent. Since peaking in 1991, the death rate from cancer has fallen by 20 percent; and death from HIV/AIDS fell more than 70 percent from its high point in the mid-1990s. A 2007 study reported in *Health Affairs* found that hypertensive medicines prevented 86,000 premature deaths from cardiovascular disease in 2001 alone, while helping more than 800,000 people avoid hospitalization.[48]

I know some who lament the loss of innocence and strict sexual mores in America today, and wish we'd return to an earlier era. However, what man on Cialis or Viagra would go back if it meant giving up those pills? And what woman would go back for ... really, any reason ... but especially if it meant giving up birth control pills? (Those didn't come along until 1960.)

It's no accident that many of the recent breakthroughs in medical history came about in the United States, where competition spurred by the free market led people and organizations to so many discoveries and innovations. (Thank you, business of medicine.) For all their problems, health insurance companies and the Centers for Medicare and Medicaid Services (a.k.a. third-party payers) have played a crucial positive role by making health care accessible to patients where it wasn't in the past.

Without the business side of medicine acting as a driver to advance science, we'd be thrown back into the kinds of health outcomes we had in the 1930s and 1940s. Back then, if you had a pain in your chest, you didn't go to the doctor because you couldn't afford it, and what could they really do for you anyway? So you lived with it until you dropped dead. Without insurers, without the federal government, without drug companies and technology companies, we'd be facing a moral and mortal catastrophe.

This was on my mind about a year ago, when I sat with some of the most influential CEOs in health care on a panel at the University of Miami: the CEO of the American Medical Association, James Madara; the CEO of the American Hospital Association, Richard Pollack; the CEO of America's Health Insurance Plans and former head of the Centers for Medicare and Medicaid Services, Marilyn Tavenner; and the president and CEO of the Healthcare Financial Management Association, Joe Fifer. And of course me, Halee Fischer-Wright, CEO of Medical Group Management Association.

As I sat in my blue suit, listening to all the other CEOs in their blue suits, it dawned on me that even though we all had different perspectives and different values, we all had one thing in common. We agreed on the outcomes we wanted: cost-effective, high-quality medical care that leads to high patient satisfaction. (They give you a CEO handbook with words like that after they teach you the secret handshake.) And that agreement holds true for almost every player in health care, I believe. However, we all pursue those lauded goals with our own motivations and industry pressures.

Take Philip Mason's case, for instance. For all the praise that Sovaldi has rightfully received for saving Philip's life and the lives of many others, there's been just one rather glaring problem: the small yellow pill costs $1,000—for *each* pill. When he was taking Sovaldi, Philip had no idea that the full twelve-week course of treatment would cost $84,000, plus the expense of the companion medication—which, thankfully, was covered by a combination of his insurance company, public assistance plans, and the manufacturer itself.

78

When Gilead announced the price of the drug in 2013, public outrage was swift, prompting angry reactions from pretty much everyone—health insurance companies, patient advocates, the Centers for Medicare and Medicaid, hospitals, physicians, and pharmacy benefit organizations. The strain it placed on state health budgets prompted one well-known health advocate to call it "the drug that is bankrupting America."

Most people go into medicine because they want to make a difference and benefit others. Patients seek health care when they're sick and possibly vulnerable. And where providers and patients meet, cynicism tends to arise about the motivations of those running the business side of medicine—especially when a lifesaving treatment costs an arm and a leg.

Is this cynicism understandable? Sure.

But applying moralistic judgments of "good" or "bad" to the motivations of businesspeople prevents providers and patients from being able to work together to transform the health-care system in ways that could prove beneficial for all of us—business included. Yes, some business decisions are made to leverage financial success. That is, by definition, the nature of business. Finding fault with the need to make a profit will only make us lose ground as we try to communicate our needs to the business community.

If we foster an adversarial relationship with the business side of medicine and refuse to speak its language, how will we get around to using its lever arm for change?

Original Sin and the Loss of Trust

Here's a little fun fact about health care: Whenever talk turns to the business of medicine, eventually the road leads back to President Richard Nixon. Of all the White House conversations secretly recorded by Nixon, the brief exchange he had in the Oval Office with White House counsel and Assistant to the President for Domestic Affairs John Ehrlichman on February 17, 1971, doesn't quite rise

79

to the level of the infamous 1972 tape with the eighteen-and-a-half-minute gap in which Nixon allegedly discussed Watergate. But for those who wonder how we got where we are today on the business of medicine, the conversation provides a candid glimpse at the rise of business as an entity in medicine—one that took control away from the people wearing stethoscopes and handed it over to the people wearing eyeshades (which my accountant mother likes to remind us is how we used to describe the "people who pay the bills").

Nixon had proposed a new health-care strategy based on health maintenance, an approach pioneered by the California-based Kaiser Permanente health system, which provided basic health services to its members in exchange for a flat fee. The idea was to curb health costs by emphasizing preventive care to avoid more costly sick care—an idea we have been rehashing as a nation ever since.

But as revealed in the secret Nixon tapes—recorded less than twenty-four hours before he submitted his new health strategy to Congress—something more cynical was driving Nixon's policies. On the tape, Nixon admits his uncertainty about "these health-care maintenance organizations," and Ehrlichman reassures him. "I had Edgar Kaiser come in," Ehrlichman says, "and the reason he can do it … is because all of the incentives are toward less medical care, because—the less care they give them, the more money they make." Nixon's conclusion? "Not bad."

Now, did Ehrlichman accurately represent Kaiser's comments? Well, since you asked, the answer is no, not really: what Ehrlichman *didn't* share with the president was that the focus of Kaiser Permanente (then and now) was keeping people healthy—and that keeping people healthy is a very effective way of decreasing the costs of providing health care. In fact, it's a great way to do business.

And in all fairness to President Nixon, he had reason to be concerned about costs in 1971. Just six years earlier, his predecessor, President Lyndon B. Johnson, had passed into law two federal health programs: one, called Medicare, paid for health care for senior citizens; the other, called Medicaid, helped pay for health care for people living in poverty or with a disability. Both were important: Until Medicare, more than half of all seniors either went without health care, had to beg family members for help, or died early.

Most physicians fell in line with the new law. The administration praised it as a complete success. "The various participants in this vast program with its complex relationships have performed their parts in a spirit of cooperation and understanding," wrote Robert Ball, the commissioner of Social Security, in a bulletin on the one-year anniversary of the implementation of Medicare.

As criticism and praise both began to fade, though, spending rose and physicians and hospitals profited. Naturally, more people sought care once it was paid for. New hospitals were built because federal programs subsidized their construction. It was a little bit like the Wild West: Hospitals and physicians were free to treat however they wanted and charge whatever they wanted, and they got paid enough to more than cover their costs. (You read that part right—*more* than cover their costs.) In these generous circumstances, Medicare and Medicaid spending rose 113 percent by 1971.[49] Physician pay rose, too: from about $50,000 in 1940 to $250,000 in 1970, at precisely the moment Michael Crichton wrote *Five Patients*, his book on the loss of the art of medicine at the expense of business. All told, in the 1,800 days that followed the implementation of the new national insurance for the elderly and the poor, America's health-care tab erupted from $46 billion to $83 billion.

The temptation to capture as much of the flow as possible was too enticing for some. It took only three years for accounts of widespread fraud and abuse to pour in. The first Senate hearings on the topic were held in July of 1969. In one case, a group of physicians in Chicago couldn't document 129 of 747 claims for follow-up visits. In another, one doctor claimed to see 54 patients at a nursing home 4,560 times—an average of over 80 visits each.[50]

The bad behavior of some brought on the very interference

from government into medicine that physicians had fought since the early years of the twentieth century.

In 1973, President Nixon signed the Health Maintenance Organization Act, which eliminated barriers to establishing more HMOs and provided federal funding for them, too. The HMO Act required employers with more than twenty-five employees who offered an insurance plan to also offer the option of an HMO. And we were off on another merry-go-round in health care: The rise of HMOs meant a new business environment for physicians and medical practices, and new kinds of pressure on the payment for care and on the way it was delivered.

Physicians helped usher in the era of managed health because some among them exploited the Medicare system. And anxiety over the costs of health care to both individuals and society brought about a change in the rules for how medicine could be practiced. New levels of financial accountability were put into place. Doctors and hospitals were expected to control costs, and their medical decisions were subject to review by committees, state and federal agencies, insurers, and even investors. At the same time, it was expected that medicine would continue its scientific advancements and deliver ever better outcomes for patients.

With every area of medicine expected to learn the choreography of a new methodology of practice and dance to a tempo set by business, one partner unfortunately fell out of step. You can guess who: the art of medicine—the one who's more of an improvisational artist.

What did doctors do? Some pulled back from the business of medicine and began to see it as an adversary. Others got pushed out, under attack from payers and regulators.

Sadly, the advocates for the art no longer had a voice in the most important conversations about the business of health care in America.

This divide has never been healed and has only widened over the years. Consequently, it's difficult for many in medicine to imagine a future in which good art and good business have equal footing—or even communicate well.

Do You Speak Business or Art?

I took enough high school and college Spanish to get through a carefully scripted conversation, provided the only topics were my love of paella and soccer. Yet I was led to believe that I could speak the language because I had a small vocabulary and understood the grammatical rules. I held on to that belief until a few years later, when I was working in an ER where Spanish was the primary language spoken. There, I was ashamed to admit I didn't know a darn thing; although I understood a few words, I was nowhere near fluent in the language. Because of this, after a while I began to feel frustrated and isolated, and as though I wasn't doing a good job with my patients. My days stretched on forever because I wasn't able to impart what my patients needed to know from me. Ultimately I had a choice: Learn the language or go elsewhere.

Thank you, Berlitz and Rosetta Stone, two companies that make conversational Spanish attainable.

That frustration and isolation I felt is precisely what many in health care experience today when trying to comprehend "biz speak." I think of a colleague who is on the board of advisors for a major health insurance company, who told me about a conference call he had recently. The leaders from the insurer asked how medical practices would use the resources they saved if the company invested in reducing their "administrative burden" (something that we'll get into later in this book). If you are the administrator of a practice or a doctor or nurse, you may feel a little outraged that they even asked the question. One provider on the call chose to enlighten the insurance company by explaining that she would do more to coordinate care for her most vulnerable patients and spend more time with as many as she could.

The insurance leaders were speaking one language; the provider was speaking another. What made them foreign to each other? Well, the root question from the language of business is "How do we make more money?" Whereas the root question from the language of art is "How do we heal patients?"

No doubt those business leaders expected to hear how the medical practices represented on the panel would invest cost savings in becoming more profitable. But what do medical providers really want more of? Study after study of physicians say it's what they value most: time.

Many of us who came to the profession imagining that we'd be Philip Chandler or Doug Ross or Meredith Grey—depending on whether you came of age in the era of *St. Elsewhere*, *ER*, or *Grey's Anatomy*—are in many ways disillusioned and difficult due to this conflict. You see, insurance companies and the federal government mostly pay what they pay given how sick the patient is and what tests or procedures were done. How long the doctor spent with a patient doesn't figure into that equation. And payers decide how much will be earned for each activity billed.

Every medical practice is a business and therefore needs to pay for all the things that any other business needs to pay for—namely rent, utilities, employee insurance, computers, and of course staff. But there are also many things federal and state governments require a medical practice to pay for—advanced technology systems, for instance (which must be constantly upgraded, by the way).

Given that most practices operate with a meager profit margin of 3 to 5 percent, every billable dollar counts. (Just for comparison, pharmaceutical companies regularly have profit margins higher than 50 percent.) Four more patients per doctor per day can make a huge difference in keeping the practice going. That means time with individual patients gets the short end of the stick.

This might come as a surprise: In our health-care industry, only 20 percent of all money spent goes to practices, and only 9 percent goes directly to providers. Medical Group Management Association's (MGMA) 2016 research revealed that every medical practice spends $32,500 per physician per year on information technology (IT). (See chapter 5 for more about this.) Because of the all-but-mandated electronic health records, the cost of IT has increased 40 percent since 2009. Another $40,000 plus per physician per year goes to managing and reporting quality measures to state and federal agencies and insurance companies. And let's not forget that the best-run practices who do all they can to allow doctors to spend as much time as possible treating patients hire on average 4.5 full-time people per physician—just to make sure everything is in compliance with whatever the new regulatory changes are this month. Those four plus people include nurses, people at the front desk, and people who handle insurance benefits and billing.

To see enough patients in a day to cover all these costs, most doctors (and this includes specialists, who typically need longer visit times) can spend less than sixteen minutes with each patient. Those numbers are self-reported, and some studies have found that physicians' estimates are higher than the truth. Physicians *want* to spend more time; they simply can't afford to do it. While patients are stuck with feelings of neglect, doctors and practices are squeezed in a time-money crunch.

I know a woman, a fellow pediatrician, who absolutely loved being a doctor—I mean *loved* it. Her favorite activity was spending time with her young patients and their families. Whether they were seeing her for an annual checkup, the virus du jour, or a wart, she would ask them about what was happening with their family, how the school year was going, how the older brother was doing in college, or if they had seen the crazy stunt on their favorite TV show the night before. She loved connecting and nurturing relationships. Simply, she loved the art, and her patients loved her because of it.

For her medical practice, this was a problem. For ten years, the practice leaders and partners talked to the friendly doctor again and again about her *productivity*. It became an ongoing battle to get her to see closer to twenty-two patients a day when she would have been thrilled to see about fifteen—a number that meant they wouldn't be able to pay her salary. Finally, in her mid-fifties and after practicing for less than twenty-five years, she chose to retire. If she couldn't practice the art, she wasn't interested in being a part of the business.

Again, it takes time to have the important conversations, to listen closely, and to build relationships. Often it takes a lot more time than what will be covered by what the practice is paid for the visit. When physicians get shut off from the art of medicine over business concerns, they run out of patience with listening to the language of business. In a recent survey of 16,000 physicians by the Physicians Foundation, fewer than one in seven American doctors said they had sufficient time to achieve what they want to achieve in their day. Once again, it comes back to time, for time is a doctor's most valuable commodity.

If you don't work in the health-care industry, you might be asking, "If the average visit is about fifteen minutes and doctors are seeing about twenty patients a day (total time five hours) and have support from other people in the practice, where does all the time go?" Excellent question that I get asked daily. You may have recently found yourself in an exam room watching your doctor type or tap away, staring at a screen. Exasperated, you might have thought, *She spends more time communicating with that device than with me!* And you would be right. She does—at a ratio of about 2 to 1. Yes, for every hour a doctor spends face-to-face with patients, she spends two hours entering data or managing referrals, prescriptions, and so on in an EHR, plus some other desk work. (I elaborate on these topics in more detail in chapters 5, 6, and 7.)

The language of business has transformed medical practices into data-processing centers for insurance companies and local, state, and federal agencies. When Mike comes home after a bad day and I ask him what happened, he replies with a customer service line I learned while working the counter at McDonald's as a teenager: "Do you want fries with that?" That mandated work comes at a price—a price that practices are expected to absorb, just as patients are expected to absorb a bigger percentage of their health-care costs every year. Objectively we can see the truth: That by mandating specific behaviors for every patient encounter, the business of medicine is crowding out the time needed for the art to do its job.

It's very human to ignore and devalue what we don't understand, and the conflicting languages of business and art almost guarantee that the native speakers of each won't understand the other. The solution is not to disengage from the conversation, but to learn enough of the other language to make yourself clear and allow yourself to be heard.

Loss of HeART

There's a Michael Crichtonian cautionary tale in all of this for us. The truth is, we need more providers practicing the art of medicine. But the fundamental imbalance within medicine today is leading to a loss of talented practitioners, and it's burning out the talent that we do have.

I think of the story I heard from a friend named Joan, a consultant who often works as a kind of interim executive for practices that are struggling. An endocrinologist in need called one day from Oregon, and Joan flew out to help. The practice was thriving in terms of patients and financials. The doctor was busier than ever—she was regarded as one of the best specialists in the area and her patients loved her. But she couldn't keep staff, especially practice executives, to save her life.

Joan was hired to identify the root issues and fix the problems she found. Everywhere she looked, the issues led back to the same problem—the doctor. She made the lives of the staff and leaders hell. She badgered, shouted, and belittled, taking all of her frustrations out on them. Keeping up with the constantly changing requirements of practicing medicine in the twenty-first century while also being present for patients and available for staff ground her patience down to nothing. Not surprisingly, finding new staff was becoming more difficult. Her positive reputation as a doctor was being overshadowed by her negative reputation as a boss and colleague.

It was Joan's job to tell her the truth. Armed with her professional assessment, she sat the doc down and gave it to her straight: "The problem in this office ... is you."

Upon receiving this news, the doctor quietly stood up, crossed the room to a desk, picked up one of those boxy old desktop computers, and threw it out the third-floor window.

Joan was stunned. "Why did you do that?"

The doctor slumped into her chair. "I'm tired. I'm just ... so ... tired."

The unrelenting emphasis on improved business outcomes—containing costs, improving efficiency and access, and building in stronger quality standards—that disregards the art of medicine has resulted in mind-numbing levels of complexity and counterproductive consequences. The fact that those consequences are unintended doesn't lessen the degree to which they damage the art of medicine.

Control has shifted to people and organizations outside the exam room—those who control the purse strings rather than stethoscopes. Yes, more and more decisions about the delivery of health care are made by people who have never actually delivered health care. Instead of easing the way for the art of medicine, as good business should do, obstacles are thrown in the path of caring providers. Patients don't know what's causing these obstacles, and physicians feel powerless to do anything about them, while payers and policymakers stick their heads in the sand and pretend it's all good.

Is there relief in sight? Is there a way to dance together in harmony, empowered by cooperation and understanding?

I think so, yes. In later chapters, I offer what I hope are helpful ways to make all our steps lighter and more effective.

CHAPTER 5

Kenny, $84,000, and Rainbows

Bewildering payment systems,
surreal codes, and needless complexity
are creating distrust and frustration
for all of us.

IN 2005, HARVARD UNIVERSITY published the results of a shocking research study about people who were filing for bankruptcy.[51] What made it shocking wasn't the fact that about half of those who declared bankruptcy did so because of medical bills they couldn't pay (2 million people a year at the time). Frankly, those terrible statistics were not terribly surprising. What was it that floored so many readers of the study? The revelation that 75 percent of those people had had health insurance. As Elizabeth Warren, then a professor of law at Harvard, wrote in a piece for *The Washington Post*, "High co-payments, deductibles, exclusions from coverage and other loopholes left them holding the bag for thousands of dollars."[52]

If you had told me on Christmas Eve of 2007 that only seven months later I might become one of those people left holding the bag for not just thousands of dollars, but closer to *one hundred thousand dollars*, I would have scoffed. My husband, Mike, and I were two financially sound doctors. Sure, we had a mortgage, and yes, we had hefty med school loan payments, but we were both employed, we both earned good salaries, and we both had health insurance. *And* we were both healthy and fit. The kidney stone that Mike developed on that Christmas Eve was no big deal. He'd had kidney stones before, so we knew what to expect. He would go to the hospital for a CT scan, come out with a plan, and our lives would keep marching merrily on.

That's exactly what happened—until mid-January.

About four weeks after Christmas, I saw Mike's physician, who was also our friend, in the hospital parking lot, lovingly "coaching" her teenage son over the phone (I could hear her from three rows away). I didn't think much of it when she waved at me, pulled the phone from her ear, and said, "Have Mike call me. We need to talk." I mentioned it to Mike that night and then left for a long business trip to Miami to work with my new consulting partners on a book.

When Mike called her, she asked him to come in—the next day. As you either know or certainly suspect, that's rarely a good sign.

After returning from a trip over the holidays, Mike's doctor had reviewed the films from his kidney stone. She was concerned about something she saw in his left kidney (the stone had been in the right). "There's something there that shouldn't be," she explained, "and we need to do another scan." I spoke to Mike that night from my hotel room and reassured him that it was nothing, because I was *sure* it was nothing.

He called me the day after his contrast scan, while I was standing in a Fresh Market grocery store picking up lunch. When he said, "Halee, we need to talk. Right now," I could feel everything shift. I made my way out to my rental car in the parking lot, and that's where I was sitting in 90-degree heat and 100 percent humidity when he told me that his doctor thought he had kidney cancer. The scan had revealed a cyst, and he needed to have surgery right away. They would know more afterward.

Mike's greatest fear had always been cancer. He wasn't alone in that, of course, but now that fear was becoming a waking nightmare. The earliest flight home I could find was the next day. I walked through the airport in a daze. My usual stack of reading material never made it into or out of my bag. My husband was young and healthy—how could this happen? What would this do to us? Mike and I had been inseparable since I was twenty-two years old. *What if the worst happens?* That question kept rising in my mind and heart as I realized this thing was happening to us, and we had no control.

"I've got to be strong," I told myself during the flight. "I can't add to his stress by breaking down." Mike picked me up at the airport, and when I saw him, I thought he looked like a ghost. But I had spent the flight preparing, so I smiled, hugged him, and told him everything would be okay. Despite the fear, a big part of me still believed it.

His doctor met with us after normal business hours the next day in her office, where she pulled out a jug of wine, poured us each half a glass, and said, "Drink this. You need it." I doubted she did that with all her patients, but I was glad she did it with us. I couldn't tell you much about the rest of the visit. I remember her showing us the scans and pointing at shadows that shouldn't be there. I'm sure she walked us through what would happen during the surgery. But when we left, all I knew for sure was that Mike would be having surgery the next week.

I did what I normally do—tried to focus on positive realities. "We're going out to a fabulous dinner to celebrate," I said. When Mike looked at me like I'd lost my mind, I said, "We're blessed that your kidney stone helped her catch this early. It's very small, she's going to get it all, and everything will be okay."

Until you see your husband or wife or kid or parent lying in a hospital bed, pale and barely conscious, with tubes running into and out of him or her, with a mask pumping oxygen, you can't know what it will be like. Mike's surgery went well from a surgical perspective. They had confirmed that it was cancer, but it was very early and small—grade 1, stage 1, in cancer lingo—and they had gotten it all. But the procedure was brutal. They had removed a rib, sliced through all the muscle on his left side, cut out a wedge of the kidney, and then put him back together again.

When I saw him in the post-op room, he looked like he'd been bitten by a shark, and he'd lost liters of blood. Three days later, when he was still in that bed, still hooked up to the tubes, it really hit me just how sick he was, and that maybe we weren't through the worst of it.

What I still didn't know: On top of Mike's horrible cancer diagnosis and scary surgery, we were heading into a financial storm that might ruin us. Mike couldn't work, of course, but what we thought would be six weeks turned into months. When you're a partial owner of a business, as Mike was, and you aren't working, you don't necessarily get paid. I took time off to care for him—turning down consulting engagements, cutting my hours back. But when the first bills began to show up, I wasn't worried. "We have insurance," I thought. "This isn't what we actually owe. I'll get another corrected bill in a month."

Day by day, the bills kept coming—the hospital, the anesthesiologist for the surgery, the surgeon, the laboratory, the hematologist, multiple radiologists, the doctor who was managing Mike's pain. After a couple of months of this, I had a mantra I repeated during every trek back from the mailbox: *This has to be the last one, this has to be the last one.* As the bills kept coming, I eventually realized that maybe Mike's insurance wasn't as good as I'd thought. It was possible we might owe the dollar amounts showing up on the second and third notices—which started coming with letters threatening collection.

On the day this occurred to me, I felt incredibly alone. We had been truly blessed to be surrounded by loving friends and family while Mike was in the hospital and in the early weeks of his recovery. But life moves on, and as Mike started to show improvement, people got back to their lives. Now, with this new and horrible revelation hanging over me, I was too ashamed to talk about it with anyone. How could we be in this position? I stopped sleeping, and started losing weight because my stomach hurt too much to eat.

Self-sufficiency—being able to figure things out—is something I pride myself on, but there were so many bills and the numbers simply didn't make sense. The amount charged, the amount allowed by our insurance company, the amount they paid, and what we owed didn't always match up with the paperwork we received. Sometimes it didn't even add up correctly based on what they included in the multi-page bill. I finally accepted that I couldn't figure it out. I gathered up everything I had, sorted it, and took it to my mom. As I mentioned in chapter 3, she happens to be a certified public accountant (CPA).

What happened next almost runs like a joke. What do you get when you put a CPA, an MD, and a JD (an attorney—that's my brother) in a room full of medical bills? The answer made a terrible punch line. We put everything into a spreadsheet, Mom worked through it methodically, and then she handed the stack back to me. "I can't figure it out," she said. "It doesn't make any sense. You need to just call them."

And so I did. Here's how that went:

Why is the machine Mike needed to keep his lungs open after all the blood loss not covered?

We just don't cover those.

Why aren't you covering an MRI he had after the surgery?

We never received a preapproval request.

The medical practice said they submitted it. I have the preauthorization approval number.

Well, we didn't get it.

Can I set up a payment plan?

No.

I can't just write a check for this amount of money.

We accept credit cards.

That last one was a laugh. Five months down the line from Mike's surgery, after phone calls and debates and hunting down lost paperwork, I had figured out that *we owed $84,000.* We certainly didn't have that kind of credit.

Financially, it was the perfect storm. We had depleted our savings in the first six months after surgery paying for frivolous things

93

like our mortgage, car loans, and food. And it was now the summer of 2008. Credit everywhere was tight. Our higher credit card limit had been reduced, there were no loans to be had, and there was no way to get a second mortgage. Mike was finally back at work, but only part-time (being a pediatrician can be physically demanding, and he wasn't fully healed yet). I was working as much as possible to bring in more money, but I was also still helping Mike and taking care of more around the house while he recuperated.

I couldn't talk to Mike about our financial problems because I wanted him to concentrate on healing so that he could get back to his old self (which took almost three years). Luckily, he was too tired at night to notice that I was lying next to him wide awake, my stomach churning.

Finally, I went to my parents, and with tears of shame rolling down my face, told them it was likely we'd lose our house because the next best alternative was to declare bankruptcy. My parents rescued us by tapping their own savings to help us cover our medical bills. I felt relieved but also profoundly humiliated. *How could we get into such a big hole? How could I let this happen?*

Of course you can't plan for cancer or a lot of other major illnesses. For Mike and me, the cause of our massive medical debt—a health plan with no out-of-pocket maximum—doesn't happen much anymore. Still, that doesn't make my story unusual today. And I often think of the folks out there whose parents aren't in a position to help when a medically induced financial storm blows in.

You might expect that because Mike and I were both doctors, we'd understand the system well enough to anticipate the financial trouble we would face with a cancer diagnosis. You might think the bills we received would be easy for us to understand. Surely, as physicians, we'd be able to talk the language of health insurance companies and smoothly resolve discrepancies and disputes. But in the end, the ridiculously complex insurance system affected us just like it does most people who must deal with it, creating confusion, anger, fear, and financial turmoil.

The third biggest complaint on the *Consumer Reports* Gripe-o-Meter capturing what upsets patients was "billing disputes hard to resolve."[53] And those certainly add to the other stresses of the financial burdens that get heavier every day. From 2005 to 2015, deductibles—that pesky pile we have to pay before our insurance kicks in—increased by almost *255 percent* for workers covered under an employer's plan.[54] At the same time, premiums rose.

Patients don't know where to turn for guidance, who to trust for accurate information, or what to do when they owe more than they expected. As their frustrations mount, they don't take their complaints to legislators, policymakers, or insurance company executives, because they don't realize the role such people play. So physicians and their office staff are caught in the cross fire.

Doctors don't like any of this. Increasingly, they're the ones who have to explain that treatments are only partially covered or that they can't refer a patient to the best specialist in town because she's out of network. Those who work behind the scenes in the office are forever trying to work out what's going on with insurance. And no one enjoys chasing after money from people struggling to pay. For patients, frustration and financial hardship lead to avoidance. This lays the foundation for a solidly unhealthy relationship.

The only thing that made the experience different for Mike and me is that we knew enough about the bizarre system of billing that we didn't take out our anxiety and frustration on the people who took care of him. We knew that medical claims and billing form a separate world—a separate industry, actually—full of suspicion, demands for proof, surreal codes, and sketchy middlemen. The process is so bewildering that it seems designed by a drug-addled fiction writer with a gift for dark and deranged stories.

These tales from the land of medical claims and billing do not bode well for a happy ending. If we don't fix what's gone wrong in this system, the art of medicine will be overwhelmed and the doctor-patient relationship will be killed off.

Suicide by Jellyfish

Less than an hour's drive from my house in Denver lives a badly drawn boy who has died and come back to life more than a hundred times.

He is famous for the foul-mouthed group he hangs around with and for the iconic orange parka he always wears, with the hood cinched so tightly around his head that for the longest time, it was impossible to understand what he was saying. His name is Kenny McCormick, and he is a work of fiction—one of the main characters in the long-running animated adult comedy called *South Park* about a small town in Colorado, based on a real place about fifty miles from Denver.

Much of the bad fortune in the show centers on Kenny and his untimely end at some point during many of the episodes, yet he always returns the following week without raising any eyebrows. The humor comes in the absurd and over-the-top ways in which he bites the dust. Kenny has been attacked by mutant turkeys. He has been overtaken by a bear while impersonating a deer. He has been accosted by an evil goldfish, flattened by the falling Mir space station, and frozen in carbonite Han Solo–style by the CIA.

After every unfortunate incident, one of his friends utters a version of the line "Oh my God! They killed Kenny! You bastards!" And then they return to whatever they were doing before Kenny was struck down in the death du jour.

In July of 2014, I had reason to believe that Kenny had left South Park and gone to work as a consultant for the federal government. That was the month that the Centers for Medicare and Medicaid Systems (our old friend CMS) released the final rule on something that was more than two decades in the making: its updated list of medical billing codes, known as ICD-10. That's short for the tenth revision of the International Statistical Classification of Diseases and Related Health Problems. Those in health care are just glad it's not known as ISCDRHP-10.

The code itself was created by the World Health Organization (WHO), which realized that with people in different countries being treated for similar diseases, symptoms, and injuries, it might be useful to have a universal language of sorts to collect and compare medical data. The ICD system works by assigning a specific code, a combination of letters and numbers, to the most common ways our bodies can turn on us, go haywire, or be battered by our environment. If you have a broken leg, for instance, the code for your diagnosis falls into a general range of Soo through T98. The further into the diagnosis you go, the more specific the code gets. So "closed fracture of medial plateau of left tibia with nonunion" morphs into the very specific S82.132K. Today, here in the United States, the ICD system has become the primary form of communication for every physician, hospital, lab, or medical facility of any kind that submits bills to somebody other than the patient—meaning to Medicare, Medicaid, or private insurance.

ICD-10 is a replacement, naturally, for ICD-9, which first went into effect in America in 1983. That's the year Medicare began requiring all physicians who wanted to get paid for their work to use the coding system. The standardization, CMS explained, would make it easier to resolve disputes over claims. But it turned out to be a medical Trojan horse. No sooner had physicians gotten used to twisting and cramming their patients and treatments into these official categories than CMS announced a new idea—the fee schedule. Because now they had the perfect system in place to make it possible. They assigned a monetary value to every single code and reimbursed accordingly. Naturally, health insurance companies followed suit.

The problem was, many found that the ICD-9 codes weren't exact enough. The categories were both too limiting and overly broad to account for subtle differences in care. WHO began work on a replacement set of codes, which was completed way back in 1992. Yet implementation in the United States was delayed for *twenty-three years*, until October 1, 2015. Those who wondered what the federal government had been doing in the interim soon got their answer.

And here's where this story converges with the evil genius of *South Park*. To update ICD-9 with improved levels of specificity, CMS decided to make extensive use of the provision that allows countries to modify the codes. In other words, they overcorrected, absurdly so. They replaced the 13,000 codes all medical professionals had gotten to know with *68,000* codes. That's right ... they *quadrupled* the list of codes necessary to record a diagnosis.

And that's not all: America is also the only country in the world that decided, in 1983, to create a whole separate list of *procedural* codes that all health professionals must use to describe *how* they treat medical conditions after diagnosis. Under the previous system, there were about 4,000 procedural codes. Under the new system, that number ballooned to *almost 72,000* codes. And to add absurdity to absurdity, when doctors practice outside of hospitals—in their offices, on the street, on a plane, wherever—they are forced to use an entirely different set of codes, called the Current Procedural Terminology, or CPT. In fact, there's one *more* set of codes that I won't even get into.

As you read this, you may find yourself a little nauseated. Don't worry, there is a code for that.

To come up with the new ICD-10 codes, it's as if the federal government—in partnership with medical specialty societies—either hallucinated or researched every possible way the health of a human being could ever be adversely affected and treated, and then assigned a different code to each one. The list is so over-the-top, I think it must have involved bull sessions with the writers of Kenny's death scenes. How else do we account for the fact that there is now an actual code for the "forced landing of a spacecraft injuring occupant" (V95.42XA)? How about "toxic effect of contact with other jellyfish, intentional self-harm" (T63.622A)—which translates to "suicide by jellyfish."

The list also renews the old bureaucratic rule: "Why say something one way if you can say it fifty different ways?" For example, there used to be a handful of codes for the surgical repair of a blocked blood vessel, known as angioplasty. Now there are 845. There used to be 9 codes for bites. Now there are over 300. What I really want to know is where they found the mystery writer who came up with more than a *dozen* ways that a man can be poisoned by hair replacement products. Did he volunteer his services or did we taxpayers foot the bill for his amazing flights of imagination?

The potential for extremely weird reality-TV shows associated with ICD-10 is staggering. In fact, let's create one right now. Can you guess which of the following are medical codes that health-care professionals are responsible for using and which are mad creations of the *South Park* writers?

Kenny or Code?

1. Sucked into the engine of an airplane
2. Knocked into a microwave oven
3. Injured in a horse-drawn carriage collision with a streetcar
4. Dragged onto train tracks by a go-kart
5. Crushed between two fishing boats
6. Dismemberment of arms by cowboy actors
7. Trapped and suffocated in an old refrigerator
8. Impaled by the horns of a bull
9. Bitten by an orca
10. Caught and compressed in a conveyor belt
11. Burned by water skis on fire
12. Incinerated by a U.S. National Guard warning flare
13. Struck by a macaw
14. Crushed by an ambulance
15. Stabbed while crocheting
16. Dragged to death while fixing a wheelchair
17. Injured at an opera house
18. Laughed to death
19. Asphyxiated due to accidental hanging
20. Submerged in lava

If you guessed that all the even-numbered items were Kenny and all the odd-numbered ones were ICD-10 codes, you're either a top-notch professional medical coder or you've really got to stop rewatching episodes of *South Park* in your parents' basement.

Yes, it really is that ridiculous.

Like every other big change in health care, the intent behind ICD-10 was good:

- Improve medical care and better reflect modern medicine
- Learn more about how best to treat illnesses and injuries
- Identify disease outbreaks faster (CMS recently made an emergency adjustment to add a code for the Zika virus)
- Align our systems with those of other developed nations

But at some point we have to weigh the costs of knowing which of *seventy-two* different ways a person was injured by a bird: Was it a goose, a chicken, a duck, a turkey, a parrot, a macaw? Did it bite you, peck you, or strike you? And so on. One study found that coding an inpatient hospital stay with ICD-10, versus the much simpler ICD-9, took more than seventeen minutes longer.[55] After a while, various surveys showed a hit to productivity of "only" about 10 percent. Many leading the charge for the new coding rules are calling that a success. Physicians, patients, and especially small doctor offices do not necessarily agree.

Despite our advanced technology, and sometimes because of it, communicating what happened between a doctor and patient isn't getting simpler. Doctors are bringing laptops and tablets into the exam room to capture more information about the patient. (I'll have more to say on what this is doing to the relationship in chapter 6.) This is because they need to meet stringent documentation requirements from insurers and CMS. Insurance companies and federal agencies want more proof of questions asked, actions taken, supplies used, value provided. And they want it coded and packaged and communicated in exactly the right way for *them*. So doctors are clicking boxes, hunting options in drop-down menus, and typing keywords instead of listening, making eye contact, and communicating in clear and compassionate terms. (The next time you go to your doctor about an injury from an accident and the nurse spends fifteen minutes asking you detailed questions about exactly what happened, you'll know why.)

If you want a sense of how physicians feel about it, you might read an essay titled, "The Story of a Man Who Was a Very Good Cook."[56] In it, Mark Williams, a physician, shares the fable of a chef in a small café who created wonderful meals. The building was bought by a businessman (a stylish, well-dressed man) who wanted more revenue from the café. The new owner demanded first that the chef market his skills on a website called Epicurean. Next, the chef was ordered to track his metrics, and then use a computer system that would create recipe templates and more. The chef adapted to each change and managed to keep providing delicious meals for his patrons. And then the businessman paid the chef another visit.

"Now you will need to document your thinking more precisely using the ICD-10, the tenth version of the International Cooking Directory."

"What do you mean by documenting my thinking more precisely?" asked the cook.

"Great question," said the stylish man. "The ICD-10 requires you to estimate the grains of salt you add to your meal or the exact number of drops of olive oil you put on a salad. You must follow this directive, or leave the restaurant."

Then one day, restaurant productivity dropped suddenly, and the well-dressed man came into the kitchen to see what had happened. The chef was not there. Epicurean was online with the latest patch for ICD-10 and filled with best practices and smart recipes. But no one was available to plan the menu, cook the meals, or write the individualized recipes.

"Where is the food service provider?" asked the best-dressed man.

"Great question," said the staff. But no one had seen the chef or had any idea where he was.

In this story, Williams has captured the pressures and nonsense facing doctors today. It isn't surprising that some physicians reach a point where they want to disappear from the existing system.

I've read a number of articles now by doctors who are choosing the direct-pay model. This means they set up their medical practice to take care of patients but don't accept insurance plans. There's also a model known as concierge medicine: Patients pay a flat fee every month to gain unlimited or generous access to a medical group.

By now you can understand why these alternatives are springing up. Doctors and others in health care are exhausted by the fight over medical codes and money. They want to put their energy into providing great care.

Well, would you believe that the codes are just the first step in a long trek—or should I call it *The Amazing Race*—that must be taken before a medical bill is authorized and paid?

Twisted System:
The Path of a Medical Claim

As soon as I walked into the exam room and saw three-year-old Jimmy, I knew why the nurse was giggling in the hall. His mom, Lisa, was a bit wild-eyed and teary, yes, but Jimmy just stared at me as a rainbow ran out of his nose.

"Okay ... so, cereal?" I asked. Lisa explained that she had left the room while Jimmy was eating his breakfast, and when she returned, she found him stuffing little round pieces of Trix up his nose; she wasn't sure how many had made it in. By the obvious swelling in his nasal cavities, I estimated slightly less than a quarter cup.

I considered using tweezers to pull out the pieces, but I couldn't tell how far up they went. Saline spray might help, but then the "foreign bodies" would just turn to mush, swell up, and get impacted, making it even harder to get them out. And then I realized the key difference between what Jimmy had in his nose and all the other items I had plucked from other noses in the past year—Barbie accessories, bugs, and from one particular nose, a G.I. Joe boot on several occasions.

Trix are crushable.

I made a fist, put the side of my hand where I could see a bulge of cereal under the skin, and gently ground it down. Multicolored crumbs began falling from Jimmy's nose. I repeated on the other side, told Jimmy to blow his nose, and sprayed some saline to help move what was left. Then I tried to answer Lisa's questions about why her son seemed obsessed with putting things up his nose and to calm her fears about ADD and autism.

Weird though Jimmy's visit was, it was just the beginning of a much weirder and equally colorful process. About a week later, I got a call from our administrator, who, pretty reasonably, had a few questions about the insurance claim for Jimmy's visit.

I had used the CPT code 99212 (an "evaluation and management" code used for many office visits) and *tried* to explain what I had done in common medical notation. I had also included a "procedure modifier" for the removal of a foreign body.

The administrator listened to my reasoning for the codes and modifiers I had used, and made a note for the professionally trained coder to look up the best way to handle the visit. Her next step? Send it on to our outsourced billing service. Yes, of course, there are middlemen for this leg of the journey, this zone of the race.

As I continue the tale of Jimmy's medical bill, you should know that I've made up a story in my head based on my experiences with other claims and other coders. Most of the coders at our billing service were great, but unfortunately this assignment went to Betsy.

Betsy was a game addict. Hour after hour, at work and at home, Betsy was creating, building, and nourishing the farm of her dreams on Facebook. That day she was tending the calves in her FarmVille nursery in hopes of raising more chocolate cows. (This is an *actual reason* I once had to fire a medical coder.) Betsy was distracted, so she didn't give the note from my administrator much thought; she made some adjustments based on a quick scan of the info and hit send.

From Betsy's computer, Jimmy's visit passed into the hands of our medical claims clearinghouse. (Yes, another middleman enterprise.) A clearinghouse acts as a translator between medical providers and payers. Can you guess why they're needed? Despite the fact that, for decades, the industry has been using two standardized, federally mandated claim forms, private insurers found workarounds for creating their own proprietary requirements, leading to unbelievably complex software, systems, and forms specific to those individual payers. And so it takes a special company—an entire *billion-dollar industry*, actually—to take the information from the electronic file maintained by the medical practice and convert it into whichever form is demanded by whatever payer the claim is going to.

Nearly 700 colleges and universities accept the common application from high school seniors, who can fill it out online from the comfort of their living room. But some of the most cash-rich companies in the world can't invest in systems that would save the health-care industry billions of dollars and incredible amounts of time. Oh, and medical practices, *not payers*, must cover the costs of having claims handled by clearinghouses.

Back to Jimmy's insurance claim. The electronic file (beautifully named the ANSI-ASCX12P Version5010A1) was sent from our billing company to be "scrubbed" by the clearinghouse for possible errors (like an ovarian cancer test on a five-year-old male patient). Next, it was put into another form acceptable to the particular payer. From there it might have gone directly to Jimmy's mom's insurance company. However, that insurer wasn't enrolled with *our* clearinghouse, so our clearinghouse sent it to *their* clearinghouse. (Think "I'll have my people call your people.") It got stuck in their review process for a few days before being submitted to the insurer.

The claim was then rejected.

When the insurance company alerted their clearinghouse—

which alerted our clearinghouse, which updated the status in their system, which sent an alert to Betsy at the billing service and to our administrator—they didn't indicate exactly *why* the claim was rejected.

If you've received medical care in the past few years, you know that sometimes rejected claims immediately trigger a bill to the patient for the full amount of the visit. Then, as happened to Mike and me, the patient is left to figure out the problem. This happens despite the fact that the most frequent reason a claim gets rejected is *typos*.

Recently, I had a simple health problem, but I was in and out of the hospital a couple of times. None of the claims were being paid, and I was receiving demands for the full amount. I expected the hospital to sort it out, because I knew my coverage (these days, I *really* do). When I got the second notice, I dug deeper. Somehow my year of birth was listed as 1900 and my age as 115. Not one of the many people who reviewed this claim caught the error.

In our story of Jimmy, when we double-checked the claim, we found that somebody had accidentally transposed two digits in the group number for Jimmy's new insurance plan. We fixed the error and sent it back to our billing service. They resubmitted the claim with the correct information to our clearinghouse, who submitted it to ... you get the picture.

Eventually, we saw that the claim was "in process" on our clearinghouse dashboard, a good sign. The status soon changed to "payer review," however, and then to "provider requested information." It turned out that Betsy the coder had mistakenly double-coded the claim as both a 99212 and a 99213, two slightly different kinds of visits. Of course it was just one visit. The payer wanted more information, too. Was it *really* the removal of a foreign body? After some back and forth in which I shared more details of the visit, *via fax*, the payer decided they would cover the basic visit with a modifier for the procedure. The money—a whopping sixty-something dollars—landed in our bank account a few days later.

And so ends the tale of Jimmy's rainbow run. For me and my office, it was just one more ride on the unmerry-go-round spinning us daily.

In 2010, one study estimated that a typical practice of ten doctors wasted $250,000 a year just dealing with the burdens of the billing process.[57] That ridiculous figure shows just how many resources are sucked out the door by everything that goes into keeping the doors open. That amount has dropped a bit as more reporting has moved to digital (instead of duplicate and triplicate paperwork) in the past seven years. But many of the savings in doctor and staff time are offset by the costs of maintaining the technology, and the time-wasting and cost for billing and accounting is still huge.

Imagine what we could accomplish in health care if we could extract even half that money and time and devote it to the care of patients, to practicing the art of medicine. Imagine if every medical practice could afford for their doctors to spend five more minutes with every patient. Five more minutes to listen, answer another question, explain something in a different way, ask about the family, learn a little more about why the patient won't take his medication regularly, or just share a funny story that builds a human connection.

The billing process for patients like Jimmy and me and you doesn't just eat up resources like time, energy, and money. The complexity of the process breeds opportunities for errors, and each one of those errors reduces patients' trust a little more. I know a woman who has left two medical practices in the past nine years despite liking the doctors her kids saw there. In both cases, she left because of billing issues—errors, difficulties getting the right insurance billed, and so on. She didn't call the billing service or claims clearinghouse and ask, "If you're paid to catch errors, why did I just get a bill for twice what I should be paying?" Like many people who have no idea what's going on behind the scenes, she complained to family and friends, "My *doctor* sent me an astro-

106

nomical bill yesterday!" And then she found a new doctor and started building a new relationship—for herself and her kids—from scratch.

My Co-What?

Recently, a friend and colleague, Susan Whitney, told me a story that was so straight out of a sitcom, I almost didn't believe her—even though I've heard or experienced hundreds of similar stories over the past decade.

Early in her career, Susan, a Medical Group Management Association medical coding and billing expert, had two part-time jobs. Our story begins one day as Susan sat in her cubicle in the bookkeeping office of a hospital in Garden City, Kansas, where she was a clerk responsible for bills related to Blue Cross Blue Shield claims. An older lady arrived, asking Susan to explain her recent hospital bill; she couldn't understand why she would owe the amount due. Susan walked her through the charges, tying each one back to the care and treatments the woman received while in the hospital. She explained that the hospital had submitted a claim first to Medicare, which had paid a portion of the bill, and then to Blue Cross, the woman's secondary insurance plan. On her Blue Cross plan, she had a deductible, so they wouldn't be paying what was left after Medicare, because it was less than the amount of her deductible. Blue Cross would keep track of what *she* paid and apply it to her deductible. (Sadly, if you are like most people, I may have already lost you. But keep reading. It's worth it.)

The woman didn't take Susan's explanation very well and made sure Susan knew it. In her opinion, Susan was one of the most uneducated and rude people she'd ever met, and clearly had no understanding of how these Medicare and Blue Cross plans worked. After sharing her views, the angry woman got up and walked out.

So far, this is representative of what happens in doctor offices across America every day (although most often as a telephone conversation that ends with the irate caller hanging up). But that afternoon, Susan went to her second job: representative in the local Blue Cross Blue Shield field office. Not long after she opened the office, an older lady—the very one she'd seen at the hospital that morning—walked in and explained she wanted to discuss her recent claim. Susan sat with her and described how the claim had been processed and paid, almost word for word with their earlier conversation.

The woman thanked her profusely and praised her for being so completely clear and utterly helpful. "That girl at the hospital," she told Susan, "doesn't know what she's doing."

"I've heard that," Susan replied.

The story reminds me of the many conversations I used to overhear my office manager—let's call her Marie—have with patients, trying to explain the difference between copayments, coinsurance, and deductibles. She'd carefully walk people through how each of these things changes in network and out of network, and changes again for specialists or primary care doctors, and with referral or without. Patients would get headaches and stomachaches trying to understand. I think they sometimes believed Marie was making their insurance plans seem more complicated than they were, when in fact she was working hard to decipher and simplify. Each patient has to deal with only one or two plans at a time. Each medical practice has to deal with dozens if not hundreds.

As they whirl within this spinning ride of medical billing, it's no wonder patients are overwhelmed and stressed out. Their share of expenses is rising at an astronomical rate. In 2015, the average deductible was $1,318 for an individual, at a time when 46 percent of Americans said they couldn't cover a $400 emergency expense.[58] And unfortunately, the data says that nobody is doing a very good job of helping patients understand their insurance plans so they're prepared. In 2015, *Consumer Reports* found that 30 percent of the 2,200 people with private insurance they surveyed had received "surprise" bills and had to "foot more of the cost than they expected."[59] In 2014, more than 26 percent of Americans had problems paying medical bills.[60] In 2012, 47 percent of low- and middle-income Americans were carrying credit card debt due to medical expenses.[61] I can relate.

Mostly, when those ugly surprise bills arrive in the mail, it's doctors who get blamed. In the view of patients, doctors are the ones asking for money, and they're the ones sending information to collection agencies and ruining credit scores. When a bill shows one amount, and a month later a different amount, the doctor's name is on that bill. On the surface it seems that the doctor should have known from the start the amount that would need to be paid. The comical irony in all of this is that most doctors aren't able to make sense of their own billing.

Doctors are trained in medicine. That's what they'd like to be able to focus on. As one physician I know used to say, "I don't talk about the pocketbook." That attitude is slowly changing because doctors have no choice. If they don't consider the financial impact of care for their patients, if they let everybody else handle the money talk, they risk damaging their relationship of trust. Of course it's a catch-22, because talking about the money may harm the doctor-patient relationship, too. Doctors feel they have enough bad news and unpleasant advice to offer patients without having to deliver the clincher: a hard-to-swallow bill.

I'll be honest and share that I struggled with this chapter. For a while, I wasn't sure I wanted to get into the head-spinning details of how money moves through our health-care system. But when I talked to people about different aspects of the book, this was often the topic that made them say, "Really? That's ridiculous." So then I asked myself a different question: "How do I want readers to feel after reading this chapter?" The answer convinced me to include it. I want readers to feel outraged. I'd love it if you got some laughs along the way (remember Kenny and Jimmy?). But after all is said and done, I hope this section has raised your metaphorical, not literal, blood pressure a little.

All this complexity leading to surprise medical bills, wasted resources, and rising tension between the people who must work together to make healing happen is not necessary. It really isn't.

Mike and I went to Scotland a couple of years ago, one of our first trips in a long time that wasn't for business. We had gone to our bank beforehand to get some British pounds. At some point during our trip, we ran through that cash. In the highlands of Scotland, on a winding road overlooking a loch, between one small town surrounded by sheep and another, we found an ATM. We slipped in a bank card and within a couple minutes were driving away with crisp UK currency in our wallets.

The fast and simple movement of money is not some vast mystery that nobody has solved. Every other industry has worked out a system for making transactions easy and transparent and pleasant. But somehow medicine, which is the largest industry in this country—independently, the fifth largest GDP in the world—is stuck in the same difficult, confusing, and frustrating financial approach as the one described for Jimmy's nose. I want you to feel outraged that the system is so unwieldy. Because every last one of us will someday need medical care. The medical system touches every life. And right now that's quite a problem.

The problem needs to be solved. And it can be. A little collaboration would help a lot. Imagine if health insurance companies got together with CMS and large physician groups and sat down together to find solutions. They could come up with ways to simplify the system, to make health plans more understandable, and to get rid of the need for middlemen who don't add value and contribute complexity.

If this happened, it would mean so much to patients and doctors and hospitals and medical practices, helping all of us focus more of our time and resources on healing. Streamlined codes and simplified billing practices would facilitate an environment in which physicians would be better positioned to practice the art of medicine. Compassionate art, backed by responsible business and supported by invaluable science, isn't just an ideal; it's a necessity for making the best of medicine accessible and effective for everyone it touches.

CHAPTER 6

Streets Paved with Gold
and Good Intentions

*How electronic health records are driving
keystrokes over human touch, information over
communication, and the pursuit of data
over wisdom.*

O N A SLIGHTLY GRIMY midtown Manhattan side street, a stranger with tattoos all up and down his arms and gadgets hanging from his neck approaches a young longhaired man with shirtsleeves rolled above the elbow. The stranger presents a request, and after a few moments, the young man—who turns out to be a poetry teacher named Brian—follows him down the street. (If you think it's about to get bloody or risqué, don't worry, it's not that kind of story.) Waiting for the two men is an elegant ninety-five-year-old Japanese woman wearing a stylish black-and-white hat and carrying an umbrella. Following the tattooed man's instructions, Brian stands behind the woman and then wraps both arms around her. Instinctively, she reaches up with her right hand and tenderly embraces his arm— and then they both stare straight ahead as the stranger snaps their picture.

The stunning image that results doesn't seem to be a photograph of two strangers, but rather two people who have deep affection for one another.

Across New York, similar scenes of photographic fiction are created throughout the day: The tattooed man approaches complete strangers and asks them to be photographed together. In front of a stainless-steel door, a young white Marine in his uniform and hat stands navel to navel with a dark-haired woman of Middle Eastern descent, her colorful spaghetti strap dress pressed against his officer dress blues. On the balcony of a train station, an older black woman stands with her arms folded across her midsection while two blond-haired twenty-somethings snuggle up on either side of her, their heads resting on her shoulders as if they were her children.

The man directing each of these scenes is an extraordinary street photographer named Richard Renaldi, who was working on a series of photographs called *Touching Strangers*, which went viral in 2013 when CBS News and then *CBS Sunday Morning* did a segment on him.[62] I'm not much of a crier, but when I watched the video, it set off waterworks, as it likely did for millions. It captures our deep desire, and often our inability, to feel the warmth and reassurance and sense of connection that comes with another's touch, whether friend, lover, healer, or as it turns out, stranger.

"People are a little nervous at first," Renaldi told reporter Steve Hartman, but then that nervousness fades and the subjects are left feeling good, comforted. In a book containing the above-described images and dozens more, also called *Touching Strangers*—with photographs taken from a wide range of urban areas in more than a dozen states—Renaldi explained that what he witnessed time and time again was a "physical vocabulary emerge," a sense of deep connection between total strangers when they were asked to touch.[63]

Researchers have been trying to understand the effect that touch has upon human beings for decades. We all know that a hug from somebody we care about feels *really* good, especially when we're sad, under stress, or exhausted. As Michelangelo once said, "To touch can be to give life," while writer Diane Ackerman put it another way: "Touch seems to be as essential as sunlight." But what those in the medical field want to figure out is why premature babies who have three fifteen-minute sessions of skin-to-skin contact each day for five to ten days gain up to 48 percent more weight and leave the hospital as many as six days sooner than pre-term newborns who do not.[64] Why do wounds heal faster in people who receive touch therapy from nurses? Why did those in Renaldi's photo shoots start to feel comfortable once they began touching a complete stranger—and a person as wildly different from them as Renaldi could find? Why did Brian, the poetry teacher, say he even felt he cared for the elderly Japanese woman, his pretend family member, at the end of the shoot?

I once read somewhere that part of practicing the art of medicine is encouraging the patient's own healing abilities. At the time, it sounded a little bit hippie-dippie. Today we understand more about the biology of our immune systems and the ways we heal. We know how compassionate touch can support that biology by reducing stress and feelings of isolation. Hundreds of studies by institutions like the University of Miami School of Medicine's Touch Research Institute have shown the laying on of hands to have significant healing effects, ranging from reduced pain to boosted immune systems to improved glucose readings in children with diabetes.

And yet if you've ever felt like the laying on of those hands through physical examination happens a lot less than you remember these days when you go to the doctor, it's not your imagination: Doctors in twenty-first-century American medicine touch their patients less and less.[65] It's almost as if—as doctor, professor, and author Danielle Ofri wrote in an article for *Slate*—"René Laennec's stethoscope yanked the doctor's ear off the patient's chest in 1816, and it seems like we've been backing away ever since."[66] The thing that is most responsible for increasing that divide, both physical and emotional, is technology.

Of course, we know that expensive tests have been taking the place of the physical exam, but in the exam room, it's more than that. A doctor can't hold a patient's hand or provide a comforting pat on the shoulder when her fingers are busy tapping on a tablet or typing on a keyboard. It's difficult to signal empathy with a warm gaze while scanning a screen for the right box to check. And doctors are less likely to listen for what's between the lines while patients are talking if the electronic health record is taking up most of their attention. And yet these aspects of the art of medicine—healing touch, showing compassion, active listening—help lead to better overall outcomes for patients. That's because right down to our basic biology we all long for the reassurance of human connection—especially when we are most vulnerable.

The push to use more and more technology—which is primarily designed to improve communication between medical practices and payers—means that human doctor-patient interactions are getting lost. Doctors' time is taken up trying to figure out which drop-down menu or protocol checklist to use in these digital diaries, which require that up to *eight hundred* fields be filled in per patient encounter, while also deciding which boxes to check to prove a certain standard of care has been met (more poorly thought-out wastes of time and energy that I'll get into in chapter 7). Unsurprisingly, you won't hear many people who actually use EHR software calling it a marvel of modern medicine.

In theory, electronic health records are an excellent idea. In practice, they eat up time in the exam room, distract doctors from patients, and devour resources in medical practices. One study by Nuance Communications, which is working to pioneer voice recognition for EHRs, found that a busy doctor in the course of an average year produces the equivalent of 7.2 million words in clinical documentation, which is enough to fill forty 400-page books.[67]

I admit that I'm a little bit curious why some people revere the days of yellowing paper records and doctor's handwriting so illegible that it literally got people killed. From my iPhone to my online banking to the movies I stream on my tablet, I love technology. It has made many pieces of my personal and professional life better. I badly want it to work in medicine, too—instead of just working badly. I think we can get there—but we need to start by remembering what we want, and what brought us here.

The Rise of Digital Darwinism

"Tea. Earl Grey. Hot."

I always loved the way Patrick Stewart ordered his tea in *Star Trek: The Next Generation*. (Really, I love the way Patrick Stewart does just about everything.) Maybe that's why the food replicator, which rearranges subatomic particles to form food, was one of my favorite pieces of futuristic technology on the show. I like to cook real food, but when the show was airing, I was in medical school, and the idea of any food I wanted appearing at the sound of my voice was, well, awe-inspiring. "One day," I would think, "this could actually happen."

Apparently, the day has arrived. The process is not quite as fast or convenient as a replicator, but we can now use 3-D printers to print food—and soon not just in laboratories, but right on our counters at home. Many companies have been studying 3-D food printing as a way to help elderly people who struggle to chew or swallow. 3-D might also work to feed famine victims. But for you and me, a company called Natural Machines is developing a new kitchen appliance called Foodini. Just add the colorful purees called for into the top, press a few buttons, and wait for your meal (in a variety of ornate patterns) to be printed below.

Imagine the future glory of never having to touch your food before you eat it. No more congregating in the kitchen during a holiday as the meal is cooked, no more tedious basting of the turkey. Gone will be the profligate handling of herbs and spices, the aromas of baking, and the time absolutely wasted experimenting with new recipes. Won't it be *great*?

(In case you missed it, that was sarcasm.)

The Foodini isn't the only visionary idea from *Star Trek* that's emerging into reality. The personal access data device is now widely available. Siri, Alexa, and Google Home mimic the way characters on the show could talk with the ship's computer. The rise of electronic health records should come as no surprise, considering they weren't all that fanciful when *Next Generation* first aired in 1987. EHR systems had been available since the 1960s, although none of them were ready to store DNA profiles. And we're still a far cry from being able to re-create a person after a disastrous transporter accident.

Back when EHRs first came into use, they were more supportive of billing procedures than of tracking a person's lifelong health—which is still true today, sadly. But they were out there, just waiting for somebody to come along and give them a jolt.

They got two.

The first came in January of 2004. "By computerizing health records, we can avoid dangerous medical mistakes, reduce costs, and improve care," President George W. Bush promised to an audience of 43 million people in his annual State of the Union address. Three months later, the White House released an even more grandiose pledge: "A parent, who previously had to carry the child's medical records and x-rays in a large box when seeing a new physician, can now keep the most important medical history on a keychain or simply authorize the new physician to retrieve the information electronically from previous health care providers."[68] The timeline they set for achieving this utopia of health care? Ten years. (I'll help with the math: that time was up in 2014.)

We like to think, "If we can imagine it, we can build it," but it's often more accurate to say, "If we can fund it, we can build it." And until 2008, there wasn't much funding—$50 or $60 million a year in the Health and Human Services budget to move a more than $2 trillion industry will get you only so far. But then the recession hit, and EHRs got their second jolt.

On February 17, 2009, Congress passed the American Recovery and Reinvestment Act, which included the Health Information Technology for Economic and Clinical Health Act. The HITECH Act.

(See what they did there?) It provided $2 billion to support the research and development of EHRs. Most important, though, it had provided *$35 billion* as of February 2017 to hospitals and eligible professionals to help cover the costs of adopting EHRs—the EHR Incentive Program.[69]

At the time, just 17 percent of doctors in America used digital tools to store medical information. So in 2009, the rallying cry for EHRs became "Deploy! Deploy! Deploy!"—or, as some of us think of it today, "When the EHR debacle really began." So much of the grand promise of EHRs depends on them being able to make it easier to share and process data from one system to another—something known as interoperability, a word I and others in health care have to say so often, I really wish it wasn't gifted with so many syllables.

Instead of interoperability, what we got was a scene out of the Wild West gold rush, with EHR start-ups big and small scrambling to launch dozens upon dozens of systems that were about as "interoperable" as corn chips and drill bits. In this stew of competition to get a share of the new business in medicine, regulators who didn't trust doctors or medical practices made a far-reaching decision. They decided that instead of focusing the big new financial resources on interoperability, they would focus on building a program that forced medical practices to *prove* that they were using those government-subsidized EHR systems. Not only using them, but using them in the *right* way. That program was called "meaningful use" (aka meaningless abuse), which physicians tend to talk about in the same way that Red Sox fans talk about Bucky Dent (if you're curious, look it up). Meaningful use quickly became the bane of any medical practice that had accepted the federal subsidy. Not only were the requirements ever changing, but also they rarely had anything to do with the best ways to use EHRs in caring for patients. And if they did, they set unrealistic standards that the software industry wasn't even ready to deliver.

I'm not sure why the federal agencies thought flooding the market with money would lead to collaboration among vendors rather than competition. While the government didn't mandate EHRs, any physician, medical practice, or hospital that participated in Medicare or Medicaid that didn't adopt EHRs risked penalties, so doctors chose to sign up in droves. From 2008 to 2014, the number of hospitals alone using EHRs skyrocketed from less than 10 percent to 76 percent, while the number of hospitals possessing certified EHR technology leapt from 35 percent in 2011 to 97 percent in 2014.[70] But when every vendor is scrambling to develop a product that will earn them their hearty share of $18 billion, nobody is interested in making their product compatible with others.

The flood of money, involvement of regulators, and push for "meaningful use" at all costs and as fast as possible have brought on EHR designs that put loads of pressure on the art of medicine.

Case in point: Margalit Gur-Arie was an EHR software engineer at a relatively small EHR developer. In 2007, she, like other engineers, did everything she'd been taught to do to create a strong user interface. She talked to doctors about what they needed and wanted. She observed them in practice. She read the relevant studies. But one day, in a small family medicine practice, she finally began to understand the rise of complaints about EHRs from doctors, when "a kind and wise physician offered me a chance to play doctor." Margalit took control of his brand-new tablet, sat on his rolling stool, and prepared to do another live demo, which she had done hundreds of times before, "to showcase the ease of use and uncanny abilities of the EHR to simplify the most onerous tasks." But as soon as the doctor began behaving like a real patient, things went haywire for Margalit.

> I couldn't keep up. I couldn't find the right templates fast enough. I couldn't find the right boxes to click on. I tried typing in the "versatile" text box. I am a lousy typist. I tried to write stuff down with the stylus in the "strategically located" handwriting recognition box. I kept making mistakes and couldn't erase anything. I tried to type code words for completing the note later. My head was down and I

was nervously fumbling with the stylus and the tablet keyboard, and my rolling stool kept moving unexpectedly. I would have killed for a pencil and a piece of paper. I finally looked up in total defeat and saw the good doctor's kind smile. "Now you get it." Indeed.[71]

In her honest article, Gur-Arie reminds readers of wisdom made popular by Clayton Christensen, an expert on innovation. The jobs-to-be-done theory of innovation says that people buy or "hire" a product to get a job done. If you understand that job very well, including the human motivations and goals that drive it, you can design a great product that makes doing the job easier and makes the results of the job better. I think health tech innovators are only beginning to understand the real job that doctors need to do—not the job that regulators or payers say they should be doing—when they sit in an exam room with a patient.

Regarding EHRs, all that mattered for years was meeting the minimum requirements to qualify as a "certified" system. What we're left with, after patchwork fixes for software full of bugs, are mind-numbingly complex yet clunky systems and no incentive for the biggest vendors with the greatest market share to do much to improve them. (Most practices choose to adopt *some* system if they want to accept Medicare or Medicaid patients—if they don't, they face a financial penalty—so they'll probably go with the most widespread. What usually pushes companies to make better products is concern about their top line or bottom line, and there isn't much concern about either of those at the major EHR vendors.)

Margalit's experience in the doctor's office happened in 2006. It could easily have happened in 2017. In one study published in 2014, researchers found that in a community hospital emergency room, physicians spent 43 percent of their time on data entry. They tracked the number of mouse clicks as well, and found that it reached almost 4,000 clicks *per physician* in one ten-hour shift.[72] Another study found that students in internal medicine at Stanford spend an average of 6.9 hours per shift logged into a computer— meaning they spend two-thirds of their day on something other than caring for patients.[73] The drain on mental energy from that level of hunting and clicking is intense. Instead of falling asleep and having stress dreams about gory wounds or dire diseases, doctors are having nightmares about clicking the wrong options or opening the wrong patient record. And for the privilege of working with a tool that doesn't meet their needs and causes immense frustration for all involved, including patients, the average practice, according to Medical Group Management Association research, now pays $32,500 per physician for IT costs every year.

If only these companies and the regulators that "motivate" them would watch *Star Trek* again. What made it such a popular show (consistently in the top ten in terms of viewers) with a cultish following was not the cool futuristic technology. For the most part, that was just background. What drew us in was the human stories of care, compassion, and ethical treatment of others. That's what doctors are trying to achieve, after all.

The Human Connection Barrier

A middle-aged woman is lying on a cold, hard slab with electrodes stuck to her skin. She knows that any minute now, she will be shocked and feel a sudden burst of pain. Her body is tense, her breathing fast, her heart rate rapid. She is under a lot of stress, even though she's a willing participant in an experiment about stress response. A functional magnetic resonance image (fMRI) reveals her brain patterns. The parts of the brain aligned with her body's threat response are brightly lit.

Later that day, another woman undergoes the same unpleasant experiment, but this woman has an advantage. Her husband stands near her and holds her hand. The woman knows that a shock and pain are coming, but the images of her brain are quite different. The threat response centers aren't nearly as bright. She's calmer, less frightened, and her biology shows it.

The simple act of holding the hand of somebody who we believe cares about us dramatically changes how stress affects us. In fact, the functional MRIs showed that even holding the hand of a complete stranger had a mild calming, reassuring effect compared to no hand-holding at all. These women were part of a study to help pin down the effect of touch, and the researchers certainly provided support for an idea that has interested a growing body of researchers: Touch aids healing by reducing our stress response.[74]

Researchers at Ohio State University found that psychological stress can heighten the level of hormones in the blood that, like a detour sign, reroute the delivery of wound-healing cytokines away from the site of an injury. They also found that injured married patients took at least two days longer to heal from a wound if they had been in an argument with their loved one. By contrast, couples who didn't fight healed 40 percent faster. Remember to use that fact the next time your spouse tries to start an argument over whether your Friday-night movie should be *The Princess Bride* or *Fast & Furious 6*.

Both the emotional and social aspects of touch are linked to physical sensations in ways that we are still working to understand. In 2012, researchers measured the brain waves of straight men shown a video of what they believed were men and women touching their leg. Each participant rated the touch of women as more pleasant than that of a man, which the brain scan confirmed: The region of the brain known as the primary somatosensory cortex lit up more at the touch of a woman.

But here's an ending you didn't see coming, and neither did they: The videos were fake. Men never touched their legs—it was always women.

As reported in *Psychology Today*, researchers were startled by the results, because that part of the brain was thought to be influenced only by the physical sensation of touch, not by emotional and social elements surrounding the sensation.[75] In other words, your brain's response is activated not just by mere touch; it's further *influenced by your expectations and social evaluation of the person touching you.*

Which explains why patients who visit the doctor with the expectation of being empathized with, listened to, and touched by healing hands but instead find themselves untouched and competing with a computer screen for attention feel less cared for than those who do experience those cornerstones of the art of medicine.

When I was in my first year of medical school, I had a professor who had a really entertaining way of teaching students about the sympathetic nervous system, or SNS, which is the system that goes into overdrive during stress. Like every other part of the human body, it took millions of years to develop. The teacher used to ask us to imagine the experience of our earliest ancestors, for whom that system most likely wasn't present. In my mind, his prompting cued up an endless series of awkward first-date scenarios, with my SNS running through a sequence similar to that of our earliest ancestors staring motionless as a series of horrible beasts ran straight at them and then devoured them. My ancestor and I came to the same conclusion: RUN! Granted, "sympathetic" might seem like the wrong name for it, given that it's the system governing fight or flight. When something triggers the SNS, it signals the release of stress hormones, adrenaline and cortisol, which cause your heart rate to jump, your muscles to tighten, and your blood pressure to rise. This is what our brain developed to save our ancestors from the hungry beasts chasing them, and in the short term, it can help you run faster, jump higher, and fight harder. But stress hormones aren't at all good for you in the long term, especially when you're already sick or wounded.

Chronic stress has been linked to all sorts of nasty health issues, and cortisol has earned the very bad sobriquet of "the death hormone." Of course, without cortisol, we would also be dead, because we'd never get up in the morning. But physicians and researchers have learned the importance of keeping the whole stress response under control, *especially* when we have a lot of healing that needs to be done. Because when the SNS is in high gear for too long, our immune system suffers, and we aren't well protected against infection. When fight or flight really gets going, our ability to repair tissue and heal wounds is in jeopardy—because when you're running from a hungry tiger, the body's priority is getting you to safety, not putting energy into tending your wounds.

Unfortunately, being sick is pretty stressful, and being chronically sick can be chronically stressful. The body doesn't sift out whether to go into fight or flight, depending on whether the stress occurs in a bedridden patient or in someone running from a mountain lion; the body takes its cues from the brain. That is why there's a need to convince the brain that it's okay to calm down, and why the role that healers can play in reducing stress is so crucial.

What can they do? Well, as we've seen, touch helps calm the SNS. Touch opens up the physical vocabulary of caring seen at the beginning of this chapter, and soothes a patient's distress. The more that patients feel cared for, the more their stress response goes down. All forms of tender loving care (TLC), such as showing compassion, listening attentively, and communicating with empathy have been proven to help—even just looking a patient in the eye helps. One study of patients proved (although I'm not sure it really needed to be proved) that the more time the doctor spent actually looking at the patient, the more the patient felt connected to and empathy from the doctor, and the more the patient liked the doctor.[76] Simple eye contact makes us feel more cared for.

Doctors need to have time for TLC, not only to reassure, comfort, and calm patients but also to do their jobs well. They need time to read body language or to make a human connection that will open up trust so that patients will confide in them more honestly and fully. They need their hands free to get an accurate diagnosis.

They need to be able to practice the art of medicine.

Everybody in health care knows this to be true, and researchers are proving it every day with more brain scans and surveys and behavioral studies. So why is it so hard for regulators and company executives to understand physician resistance to poorly designed EHRs when studies are supporting their complaints?

How far along the road to crazytown is this statistic: For every hour a doctor spends face-to-face with patients, she spends two hours entering data or managing referrals, prescriptions, and so on in an EHR (plus other "desk work").[77] A recently published time and motion study found this to be true. In fact, the more recent number is a bit higher than that in the older studies because researchers included the time the physician spent fulfilling the demands of electronic reporting while in the room with the patient.

You might have thirteen minutes in the room with your doctor, but you'll get less than five to communicate with a nondistracted person, according to the study. And because of that time crunch, you'll get less than *twenty-three seconds* to speak to your doctor before you get interrupted.[78] The other eight minutes is time that their distracted brain is not generating feelings of compassion, time the doctor isn't looking at the patient to read body language, and time they certainly don't have to touch someone who's scared. Even when doctors aren't actively using the EHR, they're seated across the room in front of it or holding it in their hands ready to return to it at any moment. As a patient being treated by Abraham Verghese, the leader of the Program for Bedside Medicine at Stanford whom I first mentioned in chapter 3, once said after the doctor left his hand on her arm after examining her, "There's something very comforting about the human hand."[79]

EHR design creates obstacles—yes, indeed—but so does the relentless strain of proving that specific care has been delivered—the "right" protocol-based care. Physicians are finding that more and more details of every visit or exam or interaction must be documented. For a basic physical, doctors must document that they've asked a series of medical-history-related questions (even if the patient has been a patient for years), that they've discussed certain recommendations, that they've developed a follow-up plan for any health issues, that they've ordered this test and that. And so on. There are templates to complete, checklists to follow, medical codes to assign, and forms that need to be generated—all to gather and process data to make sure the evidence is being followed. These exhausting demands are supposedly in place to ensure that patients get "quality" care. Is that what they're getting? We'll explore that question even more in chapter 7.

And you wonder why, every time that my husband, Mike, spends more time adding data to his EHR than he does interacting with patients, and I ask him how his day went, he replies with our family catchphrase gleaned from teenage years spent working at McDonald's: "Do you want fries with that?" Again, with every click, we add another word in homage to the business of medicine, while simultaneously writing the obituary of the art of medicine.

Recently I spoke with the lead author on that journal article that discussed the frightening statistic of 4,000 mouse clicks *per physician* in one ten-hour shift. He told me that he ran into the pediatrician he'd seen for his entire childhood one day, and the doctor asked if he'd like his medical records, which the doctor had kept. Sure, he said. He received two index cards of notes in the mail. Did he feel he hadn't received high-quality care? Unlikely, given his choice to become a doctor himself.

It's true that information about a patient's health and history is the lifeblood of practicing medicine. But when information overrides the needs of the vulnerable human being in front of the physician, it isn't just useless, it's detrimental. And as we prioritize the recording and reporting of information over the care for human beings, we're destroying the practice of medicine.

Data Is *Not* the Same as Good Judgment

The closest I probably ever came to becoming so enraged that I seriously considered physically assaulting someone involved my dad, an electronic medical record, and images on a screen.

Here are the words that marked the beginning of the worst health-care experience of my father's life: "Your dad couldn't stop vomiting. So we are here again. The ER doc has seen him, and he's got pancreatitis."

"He's had it before," my mom told me.

Because I'm a physician and because my father has multiple sclerosis (MS) and a host of health issues that I'm intimately familiar with, I told her, "No, he hasn't. He's had issues with his gut, though not pancreatitis. Mom, he needs a CT scan."

That's the moment when I unknowingly lit the fuse on a powder keg of medical mishaps.

The ER had done a few lab tests and taken my mom's word that Dad had had pancreatitis before. They diagnosed him and got him off their ER board and admitted to a hospital bed. He became the hospital doctor's problem then. The hospital doctor is known as the attending physician—someone who oversees a horde of interns and residents. At my urging, my mom asked the new doctor about a CT scan, he agreed, and then we waited.

The next day, while I was still at the conference, I kept calling my mom: "Have they read the CT scan yet?" Not yet, not yet.

When my mom finally called me with the results, I felt two emotions simultaneously: fear and skepticism.

"Your dad has pancreatic cancer," she said.

Only about 2 percent of cancer diagnoses are pancreatic cancer, the cancer that killed Steve Jobs. Pancreatic cancer is very serious and often kills the patient swiftly. Rare though it is, it's still the fifth leading cause of death by cancer. My parents had a rough understanding of what having pancreatic cancer meant: a death sentence. They did what most people do when they get a diagnosis like that: They began calling family members and friends to let them know Dad was dying.

I was deeply worried about my dad, but my medical intuition was telling me something was off. "I don't think this is right," I kept thinking as I listened to my mom cry over the phone. "Those findings don't make sense."

"Who told you he has pancreatic cancer?" I asked.

"The doctor."

"Which doctor? Was it the ER doctor, or the attending, or a gastroenterologist?"

"It was the intern."

"Is he an intern or a medical student?"

My mom was getting frustrated.

I called the hospital and left a message for the attending doctor, but it was the intern who called me back. "Can you please explain what's going on with my dad?" I asked. He proceeded to read the radiologist's report of the CT scan to me. I'm a doctor, but I don't think he knew that, and I'm not sure how a layperson would have understood what he was saying.

"Does the scan say definitively that he has cancer?" I asked, knowing that it didn't.

"Well, no."

"Did you speak with the radiologist who reviewed the CT?"

"Uh, no."

"Have you spoken to a GI specialist or a surgeon yet? Have either of them seen the report?"

"No, not yet, but they've been called for a consult."

"Are you aware that my father had a procedure several years ago at your hospital to stop a bleed in his abdomen that damaged his pancreas?"

"No, I wasn't aware."

"He's had previous CT scans at your hospital. Have you looked at them?"

"No."

"When will the specialists be there?"

"Tomorrow."

I drove through the predawn darkness to get to the hospital in time to speak to the specialists. I was sure they'd be in to see my dad early in the morning, given how severe the diagnosis was. When I walked into the hospital room at 5:15 a.m., my dad burst into tears and asked me to take care of my mother. I tried to calm him, tried to explain that I thought the diagnosis was wrong, but he was rightfully upset.

So we sat and waited for the consults. The nurses kept saying,

"The specialists are coming, they're coming," but eight hours went by and we still hadn't seen them. I finally had to leave to take care of something for the conference—which of course is when the gastro doctor showed up.

My mom gave me the report, which was no surprise, and an epic relief: "Your dad doesn't have cancer."

When I called him a bit later, the gastroenterologist was more specific. "I don't think this is pancreatic cancer, but let's talk with the surgeon and get his opinion as well." The surgeon agreed and then delivered the real kicker. "The abnormality that got misinterpreted as cancer was present on your dad's CT scan *from seven years ago*."

Cue an evil rage boiling up inside me.

Ultimately, the ER got the initial diagnosis right. In fact, my dad had pancreatitis brought on by meds he was taking for MS.

Doctors today are being trained to behave like Pavlov's dogs, responding to alerts and bells and whistles and templates and checklists in EHRs that tell them what to do next, that catch their errors for them. When no pinging sound occurs, they aren't trained to dig deeper. Doctors in the ER get crazy busy, and when my father was admitted, there were no triggers to alert his doctors that the same CT scan had been done years before. And so they didn't ask their patient more questions that would have led them to look back through Dad's records, even though he had a complex medical history that might have warranted a little investigation.

Today's doctors are being trained to rely on EHRs *in place of* direct communication with the patient, or physical examination. They are taught to trust the EHR more than the patient, and to attend to it more than the patient, as that "holy repository" of data I described in chapter 3. Verghese and his colleague at the Program in Bedside Medicine at Stanford, Jeffrey Chi, described the dangers for the future of care:

> Medical students (and residents and attendings) are increasingly discovering that the first encounter with a newly admitted patient is electronic—an encounter with the "iPatient" (the virtual construct of

the patient in the computer), whom they meet before heading to the emergency department or ward to meet the real patient. In meeting the iPatient first, the medical student no longer needs to ask the time-honored question, "What brings you to the hospital today?" ...

Paradoxically, the abundance of drop-down menus on the electronic health record (EHR) and the compulsion to leave no box unchecked often creates a neat construct of a patient that can be a meta-fiction. This construct is often at odds with the real patient, accurate only in the laboratory results and other values but not always accurate in the sense of the patient's story or the manifestations of illness on the patient's body.

For a generation for whom texting can be more intimate than face-to-face conversation, there might be an assumption that the EHR *is* the dialogue with the patient, not a representation of one.[80]

In one large study of more than 15,000 doctors in 2014, 70 percent said that their electronic health records decreased the amount of face-to-face time they had with patients.[81] In 2016, that number dropped to 56 percent, but maybe that's just because doctors' expectations for how much time they should get with patients have diminished.[82] And the less time doctors spend face-to-face with patients, the more they rely on information in the EHR. However, that EHR may or may not be accurate, complete, or revealing depending on what it has been programmed to reveal, how well others have used it, and—as in my dad's case—how thoroughly the current user reads through past notes and results. Most important, though, is that the EHR cannot be a replacement for what can be learned from patients by spending time communicating with them. And of course the EHR can never replace TLC.

✢

EHRs will start to contribute to the healing we all hope for the day they are designed to support the art of medicine; the day they help improve doctor-patient relationships; the day they help patients engage in their own health care; the day they make patients' lives easier and less stressful. As author Teju Cole reminds us in his introduction to Richard Renaldi's book *Touching Strangers*:

> Of the five traditional senses, touch is the only one that is reflexive: one can look without being seen, and hear without being heard, but to touch is to be touched. It is a sense that goes both ways: the sensitivity of one's skin responds to and is responded to by the sensitivity of other people's skin. This perhaps is why so many of (the pictures in the book) project an air of gentleness, compassion, friendship, or care. There is something irreducible about the effect of touching another human being, or witnessing such contact.[83]

Human touch, compassion, and attentive listening cannot be reduced to drop-down menus or data, but they can be harmed by those things. As the pace of technological change increases, as patients' and providers' expectations for health-care technology rise, and as we learn more every day about where providers and practices should be spending their precious time and money to help patients achieve the best outcomes, EHR vendors have a golden opportunity. If they choose to use it, they have the power to dramatically change health care for the better.

After all, the modern incarnation of EHRs have been with us for less than a decade. At a similar point in their evolution, the automobile couldn't go faster than 30 miles per hour, the personal computer topped out at 128 megabits of RAM, and the Internet had only begun to enable digital commerce. As we will see in chapters 8 and 9, when we begin to ask different questions and prioritize different goals, when we bring balance into the equation, remarkable innovation gets unleashed in ways that benefit patients, practices, and physicians.

We have all been present at the creation of something that could be extraordinary. I, for one, can't wait to see where the technology takes us next.

CHAPTER 7

All the Wrong Questions

How quality metrics and our focus on
value-based pay are getting in the way
of the motivations that actually
produce the best results.

I N AN EMERGENCY ROOM, a teenage girl lies on a gurney, her stomach bloated and painful. The pediatric ER nurse and the doctor wager lunch on whether or not she's pregnant, but when they suggest it to the girl's mother, she's outraged.[84] How dare they make such an accusation about her daughter! Happily, she appears to be right. A urine test and an ultrasound confirm there is no baby, but the images definitely show something isn't right in the teen's belly. The team ratchets up their exam with a CT scan. What it shows is a colon so full, her nurse is "surprised nothing is coming out of her throat." They can't quite believe how constipated the poor girl is, but at least now they understand how to treat her: laxatives and an enema.

Anybody who has had or given an enema knows it's a waiting game. So that is what the team does—until they hear a scream. The mom, nurse, and ER doctor dash to the bathroom, where the girl has locked herself in. They send a tech running for the key, and when they finally get into the bathroom, they find the girl is having a fit, shaking and crying and pointing at the toilet.

The bowl is full of tapeworms, some of which are still alive.

A horror show for certain, but what happens next is much worse. "This is all your fault!" the girl shouts at her mom, and as the woman tries to apologize, the care team demands she explain what's going on. She won't look them in the eye, avoiding the question by trying to soothe her daughter—who is having none of it. But the medical team has spent hours trying to figure out what was wrong with the girl, performing expensive tests, giving her medication. If they are missing a piece of the puzzle, they want to know about it *now*. They push the mom to answer, cornering her, until finally, she relents: On a recent trip to Mexico, she decided to help her daughter prepare for an upcoming beauty pageant by helping her drop a few pounds with a miracle pill—tapeworm eggs in a capsule.

If you don't spend a lot of time on diet websites or reading about old-time snake oil cures, you may not know that the Tapeworm Diet has been promoted for more than a hundred years. "Easy to swallow! No ill effects!" proclaimed a poster from the late nineteenth century. These days, it's getting renewed attention. A woman told her doctor that she had purchased tapeworm pills online, which prompted the Iowa Department of Public Health to issue a warning to the public. I found at least one website that claimed the tapeworm diet "is genuine science." And in an episode of *Keeping Up with the Kardashians*, icon of pop culture Khloé Kardashian said she had researched them: "I would do anything for a tapeworm." Of course, all you have to do to learn that tapeworms help you lose weight is look at medical journal articles from the late nineteenth century. (Very reliable, for sure.)

I feel about worms the same way that Indiana Jones feels about snakes. It's difficult for me to understand why anyone would introduce a parasitic worm into their child's body on purpose. Once, when I was practicing medicine, a mom told me her daughter had worms, and much to my dismay she pulled out an innocent-looking plastic bag containing a large worm she had found in her daughter's stool. I politely excused myself from that exam room so I could go into the room next door and retch. The PTSD I still carry from that situation makes me glad that I watched the episode about the teenager with tapeworms on *Untold Stories of the ER* rather than

134

experiencing it myself firsthand. Blood I can deal with; puke and pus give me no trouble. But I have never shaken my perfectly natural revulsion for all things wormy.

Not surprisingly then, "Will this help my daughter lose weight?" seems like the wrong question to ask before making a decision about tapeworm pills. At the very least, it isn't the most important question. Yes, the data says that many people who have tapeworms eventually lose weight, but the data doesn't say why or how. Consequently, I think there are other questions someone considering having her child ingest parasites might ask, such as: What is the likelihood of her getting severe, debilitating diarrhea? What might happen if the worms invade her internal organs? What kind of tapeworm is it, a beef tapeworm or a pork tapeworm, which could infect my daughter's brain and kill her? This is a real thing: A few years ago, a California man went to the hospital with a horrible headache, which doctors discovered was caused by a "wiggling" tapeworm they found within a cyst in his brain. According to the Centers for Disease Control, about a thousand people get this kind of infection from eating something containing "microscopic eggs passed in the feces of a person who has an intestinal pork tapeworm."[85] Once you swallow that pill, you have no control over what might happen next—which is why asking those questions before swallowing seems prudent.

I would argue, though, that the most important question the mom should have asked was *"Is it worth it?"* Not only "Is it worth the risk to my daughter's health?" but also—and almost as important in the long term—"Is it worth the risk to our relationship?" If you recall in chapter 2, we spent some time with Michael Crichton's favorite character in *Jurassic Park*, who asked the question "Just because we can do something, does it mean we should?" That applies here, too. Maybe she should have stopped and considered the profound dangers of rushing forward before she understood the long-term effects of her decision—no matter how much she wanted her daughter to rock the swimsuit competition.

This is precisely the problem that practices and physicians face today in the world of quality measures and the related push for value-based pay. It's an understandable push because the status quo—in an industry where evidence-based medicine is used just half the time, costs and premiums have pushed our national health tab well past $3 trillion, and hundreds still die every day from avoidable medical errors—is unacceptable. The thinking is that if we can just find the right levers to move the behavior of medical professionals in a direction perceived to be associated with better outcomes and lower costs, the more we make health care sustainable for the long term. To that end, regulators and payers keep asking the same question over and over again: How can we use money to motivate, incentivize, or threaten doctors so that they will comply with what we say is—what we can measure as—quality care?

The challenge is that it's the wrong question, because there is no valid answer—or at least no valid answers that have come close to using this approach to achieve the results we want. The clear takeaway from half a decade's worth of data on efforts to incentivize quality is that you can't use money to force compliance, at least not if your ultimate goal is quality care. Financial rewards and repercussions, like so many things in health care, are more likely to create negative unintended consequences than positive outcomes— in this case, throwing the art, science, and business of medicine way out of balance. So despite the countless times the question has been asked, we haven't made much progress with each new round of pay-for-performance programs.

Often, when I read about a particular alternative payment program du jour, I wonder if we should, instead, be asking ourselves, "What are all of the ways we are impeding physicians and practices from actually providing the very best medical care?" Because right now, there are more than 3,000 answers to that question.

A study by the Medical Group Management Association and health policy researchers at Weill Cornell Medical College found a dizzying and growing vortex of quality measures required by local regulators, private insurers, and the Centers for Medicare and Medicaid (CMS). State and regional agencies use more than 1,300 quality measures, federal agencies use 1,700, and private insurers use hundreds more—all determined to measure how well physicians, hospitals, and other medical professionals are doing their jobs. Similar to the way that a playwright uses stage notes to direct specific actions onstage, every single one of those metrics require doctors or nurses to perform specific tasks in specific ways, document those tasks with specific language, and then submit those reports to specific places—for every single patient—or risk a variety of different penalties.

The challenge, to the utter frustration of the people whose work is being measured, is that very few of the measures line up. What Medicare believes is the right way to measure quality care for a diabetic patient is not necessarily what the American Diabetes Association or the American Association of Clinical Endocrinologists or private health insurers or local agencies want to see. All of these requirements happen in a vacuum, without awareness of what is being required of the same doctor, nurse or practice by other regulators. In some cases, these quality metrics are duplicative; in others, they directly contradict one another. Just imagine if you had a boss who instructed you that you should always do a certain thing one way, and another boss who told you in no uncertain terms to perform that same task a completely different way. What would you do if both could dock your pay for falling short? In medicine, it's left for the medical professional to sort through. Yet, despite the lack of alignment, increasingly, doctors' "scores" dictate what they get paid.

The reasoning behind all of the measures is straightforward: We expect that the more ones and zeros we have at our disposal, the better we will be able to "crack the code" of defining what quality care actually looks like. We'll understand how good we are at improving public health, at mitigating chronic disease, at following protocols that help prevent adverse events. We'll spot areas for improvement in hospitals and practices, help patients make more informed choices, and create standards for what excellence in health care looks like. And *then*—drum roll, please—we can use the results to drive the "right" behaviors in the medical profession and in the population as a whole. The goals are altruistically worthy, so it's really in society's best interest that physicians act in accordance with and then report those ones and zeros—and be held financially accountable to them. We know that all the pain, cost, and ill will the reporting causes will be worth it in the long run.

Or do we?

The effort to enforce quality standards and track performance would be worth it if, say, there was real science showing:

- That the metrics being used actually reflect the quality of care delivered (mostly, there isn't).
- That paying physicians based on their performance as rated by these metrics encourages them to deliver the best care (mostly, it doesn't).
- That all these efforts to quantify quality and enforce value actually get us to the outcomes and experiences we all want (mostly, they don't).

Instead, there's loads of proof that measuring the wrong things or too many things only means that doctors become distracted from doing the most important things. "Pay for performance" doesn't pay. Rather, it kills motivation, if only because many of the metrics are based on the insulting premise that doctors will waste time and resources and not deliver the best care unless their activities are put under a microscope every single day. What suffers most when these ideas are applied on the front lines of medicine? Things like trust, confidence, reputations, and relationships—all of which are necessary to the *quality* outcomes and experiences people want in health care.

As Robert Wachter, a doctor, a professor, and an author, puts it in a *New York Times* op-ed: "Our businesslike efforts to measure and improve quality are now blocking the altruism, indeed the love, that motivates people to enter the helping professions."[86] I would argue that the efforts aren't even businesslike. Most businesses will recognize when the reward (or punishment) system they're using doesn't get them what they want. Businesses cannot afford to keep policies in place that end up wasting resources and creating long-term negative consequences. Or, to paraphrase Carrie Bradshaw from *Sex and the City*, we keep telling medical professionals that they should do this or should do that or should do another thing without any clear sense that any of it works. We've really got to stop should'ing all over ourselves and get clear about what we're trying to achieve.

In a world of thousands of quality metrics, cost metrics, outcome metrics, and ever-changing complex payment algorithms based on those metrics, we are still missing the critical piece of the puzzle that unlocks the secret of better health care: How do we measure the art of medicine, or at least, how to do we keep the well-intentioned but overbearing and poorly executed drive for quality and value from damaging the art of medicine?

Is it worth it or have the scales tipped too far? To get closer to an answer, more of the right questions need to be asked.

Are We Wasting Precious Resources?

Which senses trigger the most powerful memories for you? Seeing a photo of a long-ago experience? Hearing the voice of a long-absent friend? Feeling the touch of someone you haven't seen in a while? Our senses act as time machines in a million ways.

For me, specific smells act as portals to some of my favorite moments in life. Great research has been done on the tight neuro-chemical bond between our sense of smell, our memories, and our emotions. One of the more distinctive odors from my childhood is a smell I've labeled "cookie-rice." If that sounds yummy and comforting—like rice pudding bubbling on my grandma's stovetop—let me stop you right there. It's not that kind of sense memory.

When I was growing up, my dad rarely prepared dinner in our home. Mom did most of the cooking, and we were all happy with that arrangement. My dad's go-to "specialties" were not, shall we say, family favorites. We particularly loathed one side dish he served often, a concoction he dubbed Minute Rice à la Jacques. He would cook Minute Rice until it was well done and gooey, and then add a bit of vanilla to the glop—hence the name cookie-rice. But nobody in the family liked it except Dad. His response to our muttered protests was always the same: "You know, French restaurants cook it this way!" As an adult, I have yet to visit a French restaurant that serves his particular take on rice, even in Paris. Regardless, when we wouldn't eat our Minute Rice à la Jacques, we'd be sent to our rooms (except Mom, of course). As we trudged upstairs, Dad would be angrily shouting about our reckless waste of food, especially such wonderful rice. (My dad remains vigilant about waste even now. Food, lights, clothing—he fights an endless battle against the squandering of perfectly good ... anything.)

Friends have told me their own childhood tales of woe: battles over Brussels sprouts, odd fish-based gelatin molds, and casseroles with questionable crunchy bits. And in response to their disgust, children have heard outraged cries of "There are starving children in Africa!" or "You'll sit there until it's gone!" I don't know how it was in your house, but if you had a parent born before 1950, who grew up in the shadow of decades of economic depression and world wars, I bet you've heard a version of "waste not, want not" around the family dinner table.

Today, in America, we seem easier with the idea of not cleaning our plates, which in some ways is a healthy trend, but in others, sadly wasteful. Experts estimate that 30 to 40 percent of the food produced goes uneaten and often ends up in landfills. Now even restaurants are getting in the game of trying to change individuals' wasteful behaviors—by hitting them where it counts. As far back as 2008, Hayashi Ya, a Japanese restaurant in New York City, was charging patrons an extra 3 percent for leaving food on their plates after partaking in an all-you-can-eat buffet. The late great Emily Post, maven of manners, might approve. In her June 15, 1952, column, she addressed the question of whether it was good form to leave food on your plate when you've been invited to dinner: "Leaving food on your plate is not good manners—and never was because it not only shows lack of appreciation for your hostess' food, but also 'wanton' priorities. Wasting a precious commodity could never be an ethical choice."[87]

I wonder how she would appraise our health-care priorities today if she spent time behind a desk at a doctor's office. Would she judge doctors, nurses, and staff "wanton" for spending time recording data, extracting data, verifying and correcting data, reporting data, reviewing reports, and dealing with a constant stream of changes to the measures, the standards, and the systems. Would she approve of the four hours a week primary care physicians spend on these tasks or the eight hours a week each nurse or medical assistant spends—especially knowing that such tasks come at the expense of seeing patients? What would she think of how the most precious commodity in health care today—time—is being used?

Here's the deep and disturbing irony behind quality measures. One of the big goals of enforcing these measures is to encourage *efficient, patient-centered* care. It's a laudable goal, and something everybody who works in health care is pushing for. If only there was a way to save almost two days of care time every week that could be devoted to patients and cut, say, $40,000 a year out of the operating budget for a single doctor ... *If only.*

Yes, according to the MGMA study, it costs the average practice $40,069 per physician per year just to manage and report quality measures. For a relatively small practice of ten doctors, that's more than $400,000 a year. Not to improve on those measures—just to report. *What does that cost us every year, as a country? Roughly $18 billion.* Yes, that's "billion" with a *b*. Sorry, Emily Post ... more precious resources being wantonly wasted.

Which is not to say we don't need to improve quality or that quality standards don't work. We just need to be honest about what's not working and why.

Imagine what it might look like if that money and time were spent on actually delivering quality care. When you're sick and can't get a same-day appointment, you might think about these quality measures. When one of your parents is struggling with a complicated health issue and doesn't seem to be getting a lot of support from the practice, you might think about these quality measures. When you feel rushed in the exam room or are waiting patiently while your doctor fiddles with a screen as the minutes tick by, you might think about these quality measures. When your premiums and your deductibles and your copays rise higher next year—and at least two out of those three probably will—you might think about these quality measures. When you hear about a community where many of the people are on Medicare or Medicaid and they have a severe shortage of practices or providers to offer care, you might think about these quality measures. You might ask: Is this what quality care looks like? Or does this look like a wanton waste of resources—resources I'm paying for, resources I or someone I care about needs, resources that an entire community needs, resources that could make my doctor and me a better illness-fighting dynamic duo? Are we doing what we should do, or just should-ing where we shouldn't?

I can tell you what those professionals who participated in the MGMA study of quality measures said when they were asked what they thought about quality measures: "Each small change made to reporting wastes extreme hours," commented one family practice leader. "We are always training on reporting, rather than improving care." Because in the world of health-care quality measures, nothing is seamless, nothing is easy, and everything is in flux. As the lead author of the study, Dr. Lawrence Casalino, chief of health policy and economics at Weill Cornell Medical College, said of the half a day each week doctors spend filling in data, "It's time physicians could spend on not rushing a patient, or thinking about a diagnosis more carefully."[88] (He may have been thinking of a recent

National Academies of Science, Engineering, and Medicine report that said that most Americans experience at least one misdiagnosis in their lifetime.[89])

But maybe the cost in time and money is worth what we're giving up. Maybe we need all of the measures we have in place to improve care. Because our quality improvement efforts *have* improved outcomes, have made care in some settings (primarily hospitals) safer. I told the stories of some of those efforts in chapter 3, such as the initiative to reduce door-to-needle time for stroke patients like my father. And really, how many measures is any one medical group or system dealing with, after all?

One hundred ninety-nine. That is the number of quality measures that Indiana University Health was asking its 1,500 clinicians—doctors, nurses, and others—to track regularly and consistently. Take a moment to imagine what that would be like. You probably track some data or measures as part of your work; almost everybody does today. It's probably less than ten, or if you work in a more complex industry, maybe twenty. Multiply whatever your number is to get it to two hundred and then imagine what that would be like—how much time it would take, how tedious it would feel, how it would pull you away from the things you really enjoy at work, how demoralizing it might be.

As you might imagine, people working in the system were burning out on measures. It meant "a lot of time and effort spent at the computer documenting things that don't impact patient care," explained then CEO Dr. Jonathan Gottlieb.[90] What to do? How about just stop? A few years ago, IU Health began to cut back the number of inpatient metrics it was asking their care teams to track. They set up a committee to review measures and what penalties or rewards they might generate in the future. But what they mostly did was ask, "What are we trying to improve?" Year after year, they asked this right question. "We want our doctors and nurses to focus on measures that contribute directly to the welfare of the patient," Gottlieb said. So how many measures did they decide could be used to effectively capture how well they were improving care for patients? Ten. From a hundred and ninety-nine to ten measures of inpatient care for an entire health system. Yes, some of the ten were buckets filled with data and other measures, but the effort still brought incredible focus to the organization. And with that high level of focus, they have been able to improve in those ten areas steadily. By choosing to measure what matters most, they have freed up resources to devote to things meaningful to patients and to those caring for them, like time spent together.

To get to that ideal state, though, IU Health had to spend years of effort and time and quite a lot of money cutting through the complexity and confusion—there is so much of both when it comes to quality measures. The effort can be absolutely worth it, but the very fact that the people required to do the measuring rather than the people defining the measures and requiring the reporting had to go to such lengths to make it viable is just sad, and infuriating. The system is broken. It is based on some fundamentally wrong questions. And yet the people forced into using the system that others are creating are also expected to find ways to fix it, or suffer all of the negative consequences. When you hear stories like these, you can understand why many doctors are choosing to avoid the problem altogether and just not accept Medicare and Medicaid patients—because the ridiculously complex set of requirements makes providers actually answer the question "Is it worth it to see these patients?" with a "No, unfortunately it isn't anymore."

The right quality measures undeniably have the potential to help physicians improve, and some already have. Unfortunately, the current system of developing and implementing them is overriding that potential by interfering with time that should be spent on the most value-producing behaviors and eating other resources, too. (And in the last section of this chapter, I'll deliver the real kicker: For all of this cost and money, the measures don't even measure quality!) In their current form, quality measures waste opportunities to improve the aspects of health care that matter most to all of us: better outcomes, lower costs, improved experiences. That's what Indiana University Health recognized, and that's why they worked so hard to change.

Maybe it's time for all of us to heed the advice of Emily Post, and apply some logic and ethics to our choices about how we use our most precious commodities in health care.

Is Money Really the Best Tool
to Get What We Want?

"This is a hard letter to write, but ..." If these sound like the opening words of a Dear John or Jane letter, you're not far from the truth. In November of 2015, Dr. Rebekah Bernard began a letter to her Medicare patients with those words, and published it for all to see.[91]

In the letter she describes how she has worked for her patients in southwest Florida, the majority of whom are covered by Medicare. She outlines the preauthorizations, the disabled parking forms, the forms for transition to assisted living. She also conveys the care coordination, the end-of-life conversations, and the hospice visits where she held the hands of dying patients.

"This is the side that you know about," she writes, "and the part that is most important to both of us. But unfortunately, what I have described is only half of my reality." She then goes on to set forth the regulatory burdens she faces and the confusion and angst that the new health-care law, the Medicare Access and the Child Health Insurance Plan Reauthorization Act of 2015, is causing. (As an aside: If regulators have been good at anything the past twenty years, they've been world-class players at generating what I like to call "buzzword bingo." We are awash in acronyms: HMOs, PPOs, CDRs, ACOs. MACRA, as the Medicare Access law of 2015 is known, is supposed to "revolutionize" how we pay for health care. Taken together, they just make me want to SMH while LMAO, while simultaneously making the IQs of M.D.'s go AWOL, PDQ.[92])

Bernard asks what it will mean to get paid only "if Medicare thinks I've done a good enough job." She questions what will happen "to the doctors who care for sicker or less compliant patients" and wonders if she "will be able to afford to care for Medicare patients as a solo physician, not knowing if or when I will be paid."

She concludes with "I understand that whoever pays the bills makes the rules. The only recourse a player has is to choose whether or not to play the game, especially when the deck is stacked against them." A few months later, she made the hard choice and withdrew from the game. She now runs a direct-pay primary care practice, accepting no Medicare patients.

For a small doctor's office, it often doesn't make financial sense to accept Medicare or Medicaid patients because the practice may lose money. Even the government believes that is true. Aside from the administrative costs of all of the reporting, CMS predicted—in the draft of the MACRA regulation!—that 87 percent of solo practitioners and 70 percent of practices with less than ten providers will face payment penalties under MACRA.[93] Why? *Not* for providing poor care, but for being unable to invest in providing *proof* that they provide "quality" care and meet all the new requirements.

Please let me repeat this statement: *Not* for providing poor care, but for being unable to invest in providing *proof* that they provide "quality" care and meet all the new requirements. Their "scores" will simply never be high enough to earn even average pay for what they do, never mind the potential bonuses the highest scoring practices can earn.

For decades, CMS, insurers, and others in the industry have been asking that earlier-mentioned question again and again: *How can we use money to motivate, incentivize, or threaten doctors so that they will comply with what we say is quality care?* And yet over those decades, everybody else, including people on the front lines of medicine, are proving that's just not the right question.

Let's dive back into childhood to understand why. Do you remember that moment of joy when you were a kid and you finally finished a masterpiece—a simple pencil drawing, a funny clay creature, a colorful "impressionistic" painting? You may still have some of those early works of art in a box in your attic (or, more likely, your parents still do). When you're a kid, something about creating art just feels good and right.

In 1973, psychologist Mark Lepper of Stanford University and some colleagues at the University of Michigan wanted to answer a basic question about human motivation: Do rewards increase our drive to do things we already have an intrinsic motivation to do?[94] (Intrinsic motivation means behavior driven by your own internal sense of reward. An example of this would be volunteering to help your elderly neighbor cross the street not because she's paying you—which would be an extrinsic, or external, reason to help—but because it just feels good to help her; or drawing a picture because you like to draw.) They selected preschoolers from different schools who spent a fair amount of their free time drawing, which showed they were internally motivated to draw. The researchers then set three conditions for three sets of children. The little ones in the first group were told that after they drew for six minutes, they would be given a neat certificate with a gold seal and a ribbon. The kids in another group were asked to draw for six minutes, but at the end were given the same certificate and ribbon—a surprise reward. Children in the last group were just asked to draw for six minutes.

After this first part of the study, the researchers observed the children at their preschools for a few days and tracked how much time they spontaneously spent drawing. You might suspect what they found. Children who were told to expect a reward and were then given one *spent only half as much time drawing* as the kids in the other two groups.

What does this mean? Creating an outer reward for something that started out being naturally fulfilling seems to kill the inner wish to do it. A less easily measured part of the study is possibly more revealing—and disturbing when applied to health care. All the drawings the children created in those six minutes were put before judges for a blind assessment. The drawings done by those who were told to expect a reward were judged to be of lower quality. The interpretation? The children didn't do their best work because they knew they'd receive a reward just for completing the activity.

Lepper and his colleagues weren't the first or the last people to wonder what happens to our motivation when we get rewarded. In fact, it's been one of the questions most universally asked by managers, leaders, coaches, and parents. In the 1980s, pay for performance—an external push—became a hot new way to get people to do more or do better. In the 1990s, though, the repeated message that carrot-stick thinking wasn't necessarily right started to break through. The idea of pay for performance was found lacking, especially when it came to rewarding behaviors where quality was just as important, or more so, than quantity. Essentially, here's what study after study has found: When an outer reward is attached to something that begins by being motivated on an inner level—like doing a good job—motivation drops. There may be a short-term gain, but over the long term, especially with regard to quality of work, results suffer.

While we were learning about the building blocks of human motivation, survey after survey showed us what doctors find motivating on an inner level: the satisfaction and fulfillment they get from providing quality care, building good relationships, and getting great outcomes for their patients. That's as it should be, right? But when monetary rewards and penalties interfere with those things, the risks are high.

As Stephen Soumerai, a professor of population medicine at Harvard Medical School, wrote in a January 2017 article explaining why pay for performance in health care just doesn't work: "Health professionals do not respond to economic carrots and sticks like rats in mazes."[95] Despite all the proof that this is true, the Centers for Medicare and Medicaid Services and others keep doubling down on the idea of "value-based pay." Why? Because when all you have is a hammer, everything looks like a nail—and the only hammer payers *believe* they have is money.

If we believe that high-quality care is just compliance with a checklist based on what *payers* tell us are the right things to do, then sure, pay for performance can work in medicine. If, however, we value quality in judgment, creative thinking, and engaged doctors who *really* want to do what's best for their patients, then it's time to ask if using money to reward or punish doctors is the right choice.

Becoming a doctor is far from easy. Medical school is a rite of passage that only highly motivated people will survive. To get there at all and then to see it through demand the deepest inner fire. What a shame for that fire to be quenched by a rain of regulations and misguided incentives. Most physicians I know went into medicine because they felt a calling to heal and help others. The income, admittedly good, was a far-distant fourth or fifth factor in the decision. But reducing the sum of the entire medical experience down to the money you get paid is not only oblivious of the real reasons that most doctors practice medicine but also directly reinforces the worst stereotypes undermining our system—that the reason for long waits and rushed visits and rising premiums isn't because the art, science, and business of medicine are out of balance, it's just because doctors want to make more money.

All of us *need* medical excellence in every area of health. It's time to ask if we're driving away the best and brightest who would otherwise contribute so much to our nation. It's also time to ask if the doctors who remain are being driven—against their will, their innermost wishes, and their greatest abilities—toward mediocrity.

Is "Check Box, Get Paid" the Best Way to Get the Best Outcomes?

"Code red!"

If you hear this announced over the hospital intercom, you might expect to see doctors and nurses dashing to save a patient in cardiac arrest. If you happen to be on a military base and hear this whispered in a dark corner, you might expect that a soldier is about to get wrapped in a blanket and beaten with soap in a sock— thanks to the movie *A Few Good Men*. While code reds may or may not exist in the U.S. Marine Corps—who knows if we'll ever be able to handle the truth—hazing in the military does happen.

In 2011, young Lance Corporal Harry Lew committed suicide while stationed in the extremely violent Helmand province in Afghanistan. He shot himself after hours of intense hazing—hundreds of push-ups and sit-ups, punching and kicking, digging a six-foot foxhole, having a bag of sand poured over his nose and mouth. All this was designed to "correct" his behavior of falling asleep while on guard duty.

The fictitious Colonel Nathan R. Jessup's monologue at the end of *A Few Good Men*, brilliantly delivered by Jack Nicholson, captures the unfortunate mentality behind such hazing: "Santiago's death, while tragic, probably saved lives." The military trains its servicepeople—using collective rewards and collective punishments—to understand that the safety of the entire unit depends on each person. And when one member puts others at risk, it's not entirely surprising, given what we know of human psychology, that others might turn on that person. They believe their lives are at stake. Of course, none of that changes the fact the hazing that happened to Harry Lew was despicable and unnecessary.

Physician's lives are not at risk if they perform poorly on quality metrics—but their livelihoods are. And while it might seem on the surface that the results are theirs alone, doctors function as part of a team, one that includes other health-care providers, of course, but also the patient. The patient just doesn't know it.

Among the thousands of quality measures that physicians and practices are asked to account for are things they have little to no control over, but the patient does. This is especially true when it comes to things like screenings, which doctors are expected to recommend. Doctors can recommend colonoscopies and mammograms until they're blue in the face, but they can't drag patients into the test facilities and handcuff them to the testing equipment. Likewise, doctors can urge patients to stay away from fried foods and sugar to keep their diabetes or cholesterol or heart disease in check, but they can't knock doughnuts and french fries out of people's hands. Doctors can advise patients with hypertension to keep up with their meds for controlling blood pressure, but following them home to insist they comply would be insufferable behavior—and none of the doctors I know aspire to become stalkers.

When it comes to lifestyle choices and healthy behaviors, doctors are advisors, not enforcers. They are not wardens, nannies, or surrogate parents. So the business model of paying providers *as though* they're enforcers is, let me say, just plain wrong. It leads to a direct conflict with patients' exercise of free will. Just as important, though, it also prompts one of the fundamental problems of "collective rewards" to kick in—even though the patient doesn't know she's on the team. Alfie Kohn, an expert on reward psychology and the author of fourteen books on human behavior, describes the problem in his book *Punished by Rewards*.

> Rewards also disrupt relationships in very particular ways.... "If all of us stay on our very best behavior," intones the teacher (speaking here in the first person even though the teacher's own behavior is never at issue), "we will have an ice cream party at the end of the day!" An excited murmur in the room soon fades with the realization that any troublemaker could spoil it for everyone else. This gambit is one of the most transparently manipulative strategies used by people in power. It calls forth a particularly noxious sort of peer pressure rather than encouraging genuine concern about the well-being of others. And pity the poor child whose behavior is cited that afternoon as the reason that "the party has been, I'm sorry to say, boys and girls, canceled." Will the others resent the teacher for tempting and then disappointing them, or for setting them against one another? Of course not. They will turn furiously on the designated demon. That, of course, is the whole idea: divide and conquer.[96]

Divide and conquer. Might seem dramatic, but many physicians will tell you that quality regulations and value-based payment hurdles end up doing just that. A doctor is expected to respond with high levels of empathy and understanding to patients who aren't following medical advice, when their failure to do so could mean the difference between the practice keeping its doors open or not. The patient might have valid reasons like money, mental illness, or emotional issues that stand in the way, but once again, doctors aren't in charge of those factors.

In a *Harvard Business Review* article from way back in 1993 titled "Why Incentive Plans Cannot Work," Kohn wrote: "Many managers understand that coercion and fear destroy motivation and create defiance, defensiveness, and rage."[97] Are these the emotions we want doctors to feel as they walk into an exam room to treat a vulnerable patient? Sadly, many already do, especially because they don't believe in the quality of the metrics themselves. In the MGMA study, 73 percent of medical practices replied that the measures don't even moderately represent the quality of care they're providing. And yet their pay increasingly depends on their ability to perform well on them.

Equally damaging, the need to check those boxes in order to get paid can lead to almost nonsensical behaviors or advice. Let's say a man is sixty-seven and has been a mid-distance runner his whole life. Consequently, he's always been a bit on the lean side, but also has great muscle tone and strength and he's in excellent health overall. Now on Medicare, he goes in to see his doctor about a shoulder problem. The nurse weighs him and gets his height (he hasn't shrunk one bit!). He waits for the doctor in the exam room, and then they discuss his shoulder. At the end of the visit, the doctor says, "We also need to discuss your weight." The man is taken aback. His weight is essentially the same as it has been for five years. "Why?" he asks. "Well, your BMI is below normal for your age. We need to create a follow-up plan. I'd like to see you again in two months. In the meantime, I'd like you to work on gaining about seven pounds. Here's a pamphlet."

I'm not sure how you would respond, but I would tell the doctor she's being ridiculous, that I'm not coming back in for a follow-up for my "abnormal" weight, and I'd toss the pamphlet on my way out of the office. Do I trust her more after that interaction? No, because suddenly her advice seems unprofessional and, frankly, rather silly. It doesn't make intuitive sense given my good health and the fact that my weight has never been an issue before. But now that doctor can check off the box that says she developed a follow-up plan for a Medicare patient over the age of sixty-five who had a BMI below 23. By checking that box, she can prevent a possible financial penalty.

This might seem like an extreme example that would never happen, but it isn't. Some doctors even directly acknowledge it with their patients. I wouldn't be surprised if at some point in your health-care experiences a doctor has said something like, "I know this seems silly, but I have to advise you that …" I know one doctor who routinely presents obese patients who have excessive BMIs with a one-page sheet of paper listing a typical three-meal, 1,200 calorie diet while saying, "Follow this and you'll lose the weight." I always wonder if those patients who have struggled with their weight think, "Gosh, Doc, I've never thought of this. Thanks for the advice." He knows they don't, but it doesn't really matter—he's just checking a box because he has to.

Doctors have to pay attention to all the possible quality metrics because often they don't know which numbers will actually matter until the end of the year when it's time to report, sometimes even later. And what they report then will affect every payment they receive from Medicare two years down the road—at which point the practice could be doing a hundred or two hundred things differently. (Yes, there's nearly a two-year lag between the reporting period and the timeline for penalties or bonuses in payments, which I'm sure every behavioral scientist thinks is a great idea.) So what is it exactly that the practice is supposed to "learn" from those penalties, other than to resent patients who don't follow advice or work harder to check more boxes.

Sadly, for our sixty-seven-year-old runner, his provider doesn't have a check box for "Spent time with patient trying to help determine if weight is healthy given lifestyle," or "Used experience and knowledge of patient to decide that protocols don't apply in this case."

※

A man is walking in the park and passes a woman standing next to a dog. As he does, he asks, "Does your dog bite?"

"No," she replies.

He reaches out to pet the dog and the dog latches onto his hand.

Trying to shake the dog off, he yells at the woman, "I thought you said your dog doesn't bite?!"

"That's not my dog."

As I worked on this chapter, I kept reading or writing stories about childhood and the quirky jokes that I first heard then. Maybe it's because childhood is when we're taught the fundamental logic of asking the right questions before making important decisions—for instance, whether to pet a strange dog or whether to push forward with a program that affects the future of health care for all of us. It may come as no surprise, then, that the title for this chapter was partially inspired by a series of children's books by Lemony Snicket, the fictitiously named, wildly popular author of *A Series of Unfortunate Events*. The website for his All the Wrong Questions series, a prequel, at one point invited readers to step into his world of "deep mystery, mysterious depth, deductive reasoning, and reasonable deductions."[98] And that is what I would like to invite regulators, payers, and others in health care to do.

In chapters 8 and 9, we'll get into some principles on how to approach those questions to get to the answers that matter—to all of us.

CHAPTER 8

The Single Source of Truth
Is the Practice

The right questions—
from the front lines of medicine—
can lead us back to balance.

W E'VE ALL HEARD the famous adage supposedly once spoken by Henry Ford, when asked where his idea for the Model T came from: "If I had asked people what they wanted, they would have said faster horses."[99] The story is usually used to demonstrate that true visionaries see things that nobody else sees. Whether the Ford story is true or not, for the past half century, when we think about the ultimate visionary—a man who saw things that others didn't see—one name usually comes to mind. He's the man who solved problems we knew we had and many we didn't. He was the great innovator, revolutionizing at least three different industries while changing the way we all live and work—arguably the most influential disrupter of our time.

I'm talking, of course, about Steve Jobs.

The myth of Jobs is that of the passive genius who sat under the right "tree" while ideas, like apples, dropped down upon his head a la Sir Isaac Newton. He once told former Apple CEO John Sculley, "When I walk in a room and I want to talk about a product that hasn't been invented yet, I can see the product as if it's sitting right in the center of the table."[100] Although he was a design prodigy and marketing savant, Jobs often *saw* those products because he literally *had seen* versions of those products: His greatest "apples" were often synthesized from other people's great ideas. He freely admitted it, saying in one interview, "We have always been shameless about stealing great ideas."[101] He had a talent for getting access to the source of other people's answers to the challenging questions of the day and then leveraging those answers to create new and better solutions of his own.

Jobs's imagination was cultivated by many of the hardware engineers and computer programmers he grew up around as the adopted son of a machinist in Silicon Valley during the 1960s. His interest in technology was sparked by a neighbor, an electronics hobbyist, who mentored Jobs while teaching him to build electronics projects from scratch.[102] There he developed the traits that served him throughout his career by observing, listening, and taking great ideas and using them to create his own solutions.

> [He] attended evening talks by Hewlett-Packard scientists. The talks were about the latest advances in electronics and Jobs, exercising a style that was a trademark of his personality, collared Hewlett-Packard engineers and drew additional information from them. Once he even called Bill Hewlett, one of the company's founders, to request parts. Jobs not only received the parts he asked for, he managed to wrangle a summer job. Jobs worked on an assembly line to build computers and was so fascinated that he tried to design his own.[103]

It is no surprise that a young man with the chutzpah to cold-call the legendary founder of HP and keep him on the phone for twenty minutes would, just nine years later—along with Steve Wozniak, his friend and the inventor of the Apple I—found a company that would completely change the technological landscape for decades.

Jobs seemed to inherently understand a fundamental element of problem solving: If you want to know the truth, go to the source. And when you find the truth, leverage it to make things better. In fact, this idea has become cemented in the world of technology. It's known as the single source of truth. Taking a page out of Jobs's playbook, I'm advocating that we shamelessly steal it to help bring the art, science, and business of medicine into balance.

In simple terms, a single source of truth is an information systems concept. Software designers and coders use a single source of truth to make sure that different systems have the same value for the same thing. Take, for instance, your birthday. Each related or connected system has a simple bit of code that says, if you want to know this person's birthday, look here—in this system, in this field—because here is where the truth of the birthday lives. That simple instruction makes your birthday show up in other places, always correct (obviously, as long as the source is correct). It helps clear up confusion, remove bad information, and nip poor decision-making in the bud.

Just as Jobs seemed to recognize that HP was the source for truth for the first personal computer, which HP was building when he worked there at the age of twelve, we can start using that same discipline in health care. Our logic train goes something like this: If you want to know how to make health care more satisfying and engaging, look *here*. If you want to know how to make health care more affordable, look *here*. If you want to know how to improve outcomes, look *here*. Lucky for us, each of those query paths can point to the same place, because the single source of truth for each of the most challenging questions in health care today is the same: *the medical practice.*

It is the medical practice where people go to monitor and maintain their health, to get annual exams and routine checkups, to manage chronic conditions and learn strategies for improving diet and physical conditioning, to both get better and stay healthy in the first place. It is why the Affordable Care Act of 2010 recognized the central role played by medical practices in creating a healthier America, identifying them as the foundation for better management of population health. If health care in America is going to transition from sick care to health care, the front line of that change will be the medical practice.

Even more amazingly, all of the best medical practices—those that have something powerful to teach us about transforming health care by achieving balance—have found their own single source of truth, and not surprisingly it's the same one: *people*. Despite our focus on process and data and regulation and money and technology, the truth in health care is based on one thing and one thing only: people helping other people heal. They do that with art, they do that with science, and they make it all possible with good business—when they are free to do these things, that is. Although the relationships between people are the crux of the art of medicine, in people we also find the truth about how to balance that art with science and business to make health care sustainable.

I'll be blunt: Trying to solve any of our health-care challenges by ignoring or discounting this source of truth—something we're pretty good at doing in this country—is a recipe for mediocrity or outright failure. I've spent seven chapters describing why that is so, and I won't belabor the point here. But this is why, at the Medical Group Management Association, we devote a lot of our time to looking at that source of truth and asking, "How are the best practices achieving balance? What is it, fundamentally, they are doing that seems to make everything work better?" And then we try to promote what we uncover. It's not for nothing that Yogi Berra once said, "You can observe a lot by just watching." We have so much to learn from watching what is happening on the front lines of medicine to get people to better outcomes at lower cost with greater satisfaction all around.

In the pursuit of balance, let's ask again: "Are we asking the right questions?" (Often the answer is no.) What we've discovered is that the great, innovative practices *are* asking the right questions. And what is most revealing is that those questions are all about people. Asking those questions and paying attention to the answers are how these practices create balance. What, specifically, do these right questions help them achieve? They make it easier and simpler for providers and patients to do the right thing. They help eliminate all of those unintended consequences I've described in the past seven chapters, consequences that make patients disengage and that make more and more providers feel like their best option may be to quit. They help reduce tension between administrators, providers, and patients by helping them focus on what matters most to everybody. They help reduce costs. They encourage laser-like focus on outcomes, and then support the highest and best use of resources to get to those outcomes.

These are the things we desperately need to make health care better. Yet we spend too much of our time talking about single solution, "silver bullet," high-level, policy-driven ideas that don't reflect the realities of how health care is delivered day in and day out. What the single source of truth—the successful medical practice and the people within it—offers us is practical ideas that actually work.

Like Steve Jobs, we need to steal from the insights of these practices and use them as building blocks for the solutions that can bring balance back to medicine. Like Jobs, we can use these insights not as a paint-by-number path to success, but rather, as guides to drive our own innovation. The best thing about the questions these practices ask is that they are *not* a specific recipe that defines how we should *all* do it; rather, they lead to ideas that anyone could use to change health care at the front lines, while possibly influencing regulation and policy, too. After seven chapters, you know that one cookie-cutter solution isn't going to bring balance back—after all, once you've seen one medical practice, you've seen *one* medical practice. But a bottom-up rather than top-down approach is precisely what we need. I'm inviting you to steal from the best on the front lines of medicine (where the source of truth lives) in order to learn to ask the better questions they're asking and to create unique solutions that work.

Following are three elemental questions asked over and over by the most innovative, well-balanced practices, and the valuable approaches they discovered based on the *true* answers—approaches that could solve some of our greatest challenges and move the whole industry closer to balance.

The Right Question
How Do We Treat the *Person* and Not Just the *Disease*?

"I'm worried about Judith."

Across the country, every day, doctors and nurses and other providers say words like these about patients like "Judith"—patients like the 45 percent of Americans who are struggling with a chronic disease, patients like the 15 percent of Americans who are over the age of sixty-five and whose health is becoming more complex by the day, and especially patients whose challenges are about more than another test, the right dosage, or the better protocol. In lots of practices, though, where the people are overburdened by requirements, regulations, metrics, and productivity demands, concerns about patients who aren't very healthy often don't produce much beyond another office visit and more advice about healthy eating, better exercise habits, or taking medication regularly. Providers and staff want to offer more support, but in a thirteen-minute visit, there often just isn't time.

But Judith wasn't being cared for at just *any* practice. She was being cared for at a practice where patients are fundamentally seen as people first, where the needs of the *person* within the patient drives every action. And that possibly added years to her life.

When her health coach, who is not a nurse, said those words of concern to the rest of Judith's care team, including her doctor and a behavioral health expert or social worker, her doctor confirmed it: Judith was not doing well. Her blood pressure was on the rise, her diabetes was not under control, and she just seemed to be going downhill. She had started coming to the practice in a suburb of Seattle not long before this meeting took place, after moving to the area from Northern California. When Judith's husband passed away, her daughter had asked her to move in. But a caring, devoted daughter isn't the be-all and end-all of a happy life (although my parents like to argue otherwise). The daughter was busy, Judith had left her friends and community behind, and she couldn't drive. She was sitting at home alone a lot, watching TV, becoming isolated and depressed. She was on the same downhill slide happening to millions of older Americans right this minute.

Studies show that when Americans sixty-five and over lose either the ability to drive themselves or access to somebody who routinely drives them, the drops are steep: 15 percent fewer doctor's visits, 60 percent fewer shopping trips, and 65 percent fewer social outings.[104] For too many, the loss of independence becomes a slow-motion death sentence that leads to more rapid physical and intellectual decline.

In their conversation about Judith during a typical morning huddle, the care team recognized the signs. "What I think she needs is to get engaged," said Cori, her health coach. Somebody reminded Cori about the senior group "happy hour" coming up—think part open-mic night, part grandma at the last family reunion, but without all of the alcohol consumption, unnecessarily messy self-revelations, and four-letter words (or maybe that's just my family). The problem with Judith's attending a daytime event was that she had no transportation. That didn't matter too much, because the practice had an agreement with Uber and would send a car to pick a patient up if needed for transport to the practice. Cori had an even better idea, though. "Why don't I teach her to ride the bus?"

On the appointed day, Cori took a ride on the E line to Judith's house and handed her a bus pass. Together, they walked to the nearby bus stop and climbed aboard as Cori explained how to use the pass, describing the different routes and adding other pertinent details. Mostly, she sat next to Judith and helped her feel less alone as Judith learned something new. Judith had a great time at the event, and when it was over, Cori sent her home on her own. "You have my cell phone number. Just call me if you need any help."

Judith did call when she got home, but just to share how elated and thankful she was. She started riding the bus to the practice for other classes or group meetings. More important, she started riding the bus to get coffee or go shopping with the people she met there. She started taking her medication more regularly. Her hypertension and diabetes became more controlled. Her health improved, and she was happier. By attending to the needs of the *person*, the practice helped the *patient* achieve dramatic gains.

There is not a single protocol for hypertension or diabetes that includes "Teach patient how to ride bus." There is not a single billing code that I'm aware of that covers "patient disengagement due to isolation stemming from lack of transportation." (In case you're wondering, yes, Kenny was once killed on *South Park* in a bus, when it went over a cliff into a huge pool of ice cream, but it happened in a fever dream had by his friend Stan, which technically doesn't count as Kenny's dying.) There is no relative value unit— how the federal government ties money to codes—to cover the cost of the two hours it took out of Cori's day to provide what might be years of better health, fewer hospital visits, and less invasive and expensive care. And yet two hours, a bus pass, and a riding companion is what Judith really needed to be healthier.

Judith was suffering from what a researcher might call "a deficit in the social determinants of health"—where we live, what our communities are like, how much money we make, how educated we are, how much stress we feel, how easy it is for us to buy healthy food, or how strong our relationships are with friends and family. In *The American Health Care Paradox*, Elizabeth Bradley and Lauren Taylor tackle the cause of our "spend more, get less" problem, asking the question "Why is it that, by many indicators, we spend more than other countries but have outcomes that aren't as good?" They acknowledge lots of contributing factors, but after years of study and data accumulation, once they accounted for those other factors, they were left with this: "Inadequate attention to and investment in services that address the broader determinants of health is the unnamed culprit behind why the United States spends so much on health care but continues to lag behind in health outcomes."[105] In other words, our health sometimes fails for very human reasons having to do with where and how we live. (I see you nodding.)

Some might say those broader determinants of health aren't the responsibility of a primary care practice (although those same practices are being held accountable for the outcomes they can't achieve when those social and economic factors aren't addressed). I don't think Dr. Rushika Fernandopulle sees it in quite the same way. "We have a population of people; they are our responsibility," he shared, after telling the story of Judith. "How do we improve their health and keep them out of trouble? How can we be creative?" These are the questions he asked when he founded Iora Health, a Boston-based national organization that owns the practice Judith visits, after years of frustration trying to practice primary care medicine the way he felt was right within a system that worked against him. Judith's story seems like an extreme example of how one team chose to answer those questions—a hero story—but in fact, these types of interventions are pretty common at Iora. "I think what we're missing in health care," Rushika said, "is that we're trying to solve every problem with a billable medical thing when we could do other, more effective things."

So how does Iora, under Rushika's leadership, solve the common challenges that keep practices from focusing on what it takes to help real people be healthier? On the Iora website, they proudly share the tenets of their "simple yet radically different approach to restoring humanity to health care ... Team-based care that puts the patient first; a payment system based on care, not billing codes; and technology built around people, not process." Strict rules and onerous administrative requirements aren't great foundations for patient-centered creative thinking. So Rushika decided to ditch a lot of them and figure out how to follow the rest without getting in the way of the ultimate goal. In other words, Iora tapped into something that has helped human beings solve problems for centuries: common sense.

First, look at their health coaches. Health coaches in practices *not* operated by Iora—those that have them—tend to be nurses. But at Iora, they look for people who have a deep interest in health, but who have experience outside the industry, especially people who have worked in the service industry. After all, they are there to serve the needs of the patient in their journey to better health.

Their approach to electronic health records deserves some contemplation, too. They couldn't find an EHR anywhere on the market that didn't seem to interfere with the kind of care they believed in, or one that supported their intensive team-based approach—where the patient is a part of the team. So they built their own, designing it from scratch with one goal: *Make it easy for every person on the team to use and make sure it doesn't interrupt the flow of good care.* At Iora, patients have online access to their medical records, almost in full, eliminating frustrations like the tedious phone tag with a nurse to find out the results of a blood test. Even better, patients can contribute to it, sharing their results from at-home testing, like glucose or blood pressure. "We call it a collaborative care platform," explained Rushika. "You just put down what you did and don't worry about anything else. We don't code. We ignore meaningful use." They also don't demand that physicians track their performance on hundreds of process-based quality measures via the EHR. And yet against all odds, somehow—amazingly—without codes, without gargantuan efforts to prove they're doing right by patients, without warehouses full of data, they are taking incredibly good care of some of the most complex patient populations.

And then there's the money issue. Much like an HMO, Iora is paid a lump sum for each patient, but that amount is generally higher than most insurers or employers are used to paying for primary care. If primary care is typically 5 percent of the overall cost of care for a patient, Iora is asking for an amount that's closer to 10 percent based on average costs. The goal is to eliminate hurdles to helping patients improve their health by making everything free—no copays, no upcharges for the classes or group meetings, free health coaches, even free transportation at some practices. Their refusal to compromise on this is the main reason Iora was denied when they applied to be a part of a program for primary care transformation through the Center for Medicare and Medicaid Innovation (a division of CMS). You may not know this, but practices that accept Medicare patients are legally required to charge a copay. Iora gets around this by working only with patients in the Medicare Advantage program, which are plans sold by private insurance companies that provide Medicare benefits, often allowing for more flexibility while covering more services than traditional Medicare.

Iora's argument—so far convincing to some but not a lot of payers—is that more resources devoted to great, comprehensive, well-coordinated, patient-centric primary care reduce the cost per person overall by reducing downstream costs, like emergency room visits, hospital admissions, dialysis, and so on. In other words, investing more up front in getting people healthy or keeping people healthy saves much more money down the road. With more than thirty practices in eleven different cities, they're building the proof they need across a wide range of patient populations.

Who are these populations of patients? They are the carpenters in a regional trade union in New England. (They and their lucky family members can take a free fitness class called Hammer Time, which I desperately want to attend.) They are hotel and restaurant workers in Las Vegas. They are low-income women in immigrant communities in Queens, New York. They are the employees of Dartmouth College in New Hampshire. And in Denver, Seattle, and Phoenix, they are patients on a Medicare Advantage plan with Humana.

For these people, Iora is reducing hospitalizations (compared to matched control groups) by 30 to 45 percent, ER visits by as much as 23 percent, and visits to specialists by as much as 39 percent (depending on the practice). The result is decreased overall costs— by as much as 26 percent. It doesn't take a genius to figure out the reason: The art of medicine is being given the room it needs so that people responsible for the health of these populations can listen, learn, and create tailored solutions patient by patient, informed by the science of medicine and supported by the business of medicine.

From a practice perspective, Iora manages costs based on doing what it takes to do right by the patient. Often that isn't another expensive test or weeks of physical therapy, but a regular free yoga class or a little extra coaching. It's up to the care teams to decide where to devote their time, attention, and resources to help the people they care for be healthier. And Iora doesn't use money to incentivize those teams. "I think the reason people focus on money is because they feel they can't control culture. We get the culture right, and then the rest of the stuff just follows. We don't hire people who do the right thing because we're paying them to but because that's what gets them out of bed in the morning. If you're not doing the right thing, we're going to ask you to leave and find someone who will. In general, that works really well." It works so well that over the past six years only two doctors have voluntarily left Iora, and they now have about eighty on staff. And while it takes a few years for individual practices to break even and then become profitable, the older offices have already passed that point, and the new locations are becoming profitable faster.

"I think what a lot of people are doing to fix health care is adding more things on top of what we have now," said Rushika. "Patient-centered medical homes, meaningful use, accountable care organizations—they just add more check boxes, more clicks, more transactions. That's exactly the wrong point. The point is to get rid of the stuff so that doctors can go back to focusing on taking care of patients. Then it feels like a more winnable game."

So what does it take to help real people with real-world challenges improve their health—which improves outcomes and reduces costs—in a way that's far more satisfying? It takes a focus on healthier people rather than a focus on disease. It takes practices full of people free to do what is right for each patient, with the time and resources to address more than just the basics, and with providers—doctors, nurses, coaches—who feel supported in their drive to do their best work to help patients be as healthy as possible.

The Right Approach
Design medical care for healthier *people* instead of strictly for diagnosis and treatment of *disease*.

The Right Question
What Do People Actually Want—Not What Do We *Think* They Want—Out of Health Care?

A friend of a friend was just a handful of weeks away from forty. She was an outgoing, fun-loving, popular woman, and her birthday shindig was sure to be a major event, with friends and family converging on the city where she lived, a large cast of locals on the guest list, and more. Her husband very sweetly told her not to worry about a thing. He would tell her where to be and when on the day of the big party, and otherwise, she was expected to keep her nose out of it.

She made one request, and she was serious as a proverbial heart attack about her one request: She did not want the party to be at their house or the house of any friends or family. She didn't want to feel responsible for cleaning up for it and she didn't want to have to clean up after it. She had hosted enough parties for her friends' big days to know what the aftermath would be like—the recycling alone took weeks to deal with.

The big day finally arrived and she was given her exciting coordinates: a street corner in downtown Denver at noon. There she stood when a Town Car pulled up for her and then drove her out of the city to Chatfield Lake, where a boat full of family and friends from faraway awaited her. On she hopped to cheers and hugs. "Where are we going?" she asked her husband, knowing there were many more people who had been invited. His lips were still sealed, though. They spent the afternoon on the lake, enjoying cocktails and the beautiful weather. They docked, and then climbed aboard a luxury van that was waiting for them, and her excitement climbed. Onto the highway they went, heading back toward the city. But just as they were getting close, the van detoured toward the mountains ... away from the city and all of the spots she had imagined he might have reserved.

And then they took the exit into her neighborhood.

And then they turned onto her street.

And there were the hundred or so invited friends and family standing on her lawn.

"Aren't you surprised?" her husband asked with a big grin.

Are you kidding me?!

Sometimes we really believe we know the truth about what people want—and our assumptions are wrong. Sometimes they *tell* us the truth about what they want—and we just don't listen. Both happen in health care every day. But when Brian Kelly discovered he had been falling victim to the first trap, he made sure he didn't fall victim to the second.

"We don't do very well when it comes to providing urgent care services for women," Brian told me in a conversation we had in Portland, Oregon, in August of 2016, when I toured his office. His interest in the topic makes a lot of sense: he's the CEO of Women's Healthcare Associates (WHA) in Portland, Oregon, a medical group with a handful of practices around the city. A few years back, he and the company's board of advisors read *The Innovator's Prescription* by Clayton Christensen, which spawned a task group, which spawned the idea that it was time to do something about women's unmet urgent care needs. With the rise of urgent care clinics, surely women needed one designed to meet their specific health problems. So the task force took the obvious first step: They registered a handful of URLs based on variations of "women's health-care express."

"We really wanted to get out in front of this need we saw, and develop a business case for providing these urgent care services for women," Brian explained.

Imagine their surprise, then, when at the very first focus group they held to talk about the specifics of such a service, the women in the room told those on the other side of the table that they didn't want it. They didn't want express, or zoom, or anything else that felt fast and furious. "I want relationships," one woman said, and the rest nodded along.

Personally, I like to imagine this as the moment in the movie *Bad Moms* when Mila Kunis stands up as a candidate for PTA president at her kids' school and gives a rousing speech about what she and her fellow moms really need, rather than being told by others what they think they need, arguing: We're in this together. We've got to have each other's backs.

What Brian and his team heard in that room wasn't unique to their practice, their specialty, or their location. Patients have been telling us that this is what they want for a long time, but the maelstrom of policy changes over the past forty or fifty years seem to keep insisting that we shouldn't listen, that other people know better. In the fall of 2013, Leana Wen, then an emergency medicine attending and the director of patient-centered care research at the George Washington University Medical Center, did some groundbreaking work to prove them wrong. Wen wanted to explore the question "What do people want from their health care?" To get unbiased feedback, her team at the medical center conducted a "street study," fanning out across Washington, DC, and randomly approaching people. Each person who agreed to be interviewed was asked two questions, but the first was most revealing: Describe a positive and a negative experience you've had with health care, including the things about each experience that made them good or bad. Of the 102 total answers given to both the positive and the negative side of the question, *every single volunteer* chose to answer with a story about their doctor. Not a single person volunteered a story about other players in health care. And when it came to the question of a positive experience, the vast majority of the people described doctors who listened well, explained well, and were caring and compassionate.

What that sounds like to me is a healthy relationship. That was Wen's conclusion, too. "As policymakers and administrators propose innovations and measures of quality," she wrote, "they will need to consider the strong emphasis people place on the importance of the doctor-patient relationship."[106]

To which every patient, physician, and practice administrator in America responds: *duh!* It shouldn't take a study to know that patients desire a relationship in which their doctor looks them in the eye and listens to them, explains their options in language they can understand, and delivers care with an empathetic, compassionate touch. And yet we're all pretty good at driving right by all of that on our way to our big goals. Even at WHA, they were in danger of doing just that, despite the fact that the patient experience and the relationship that creates it has always been a pillar of their approach, of their culture, of their business strategy. Since 2004, they've defined their delivery of that experience with four words: inviting, authentic, knowledgeable, and caring.

Brian and his team didn't do what some in health care might have done: plow ahead with their plans, sure in their assumptions that urgent care was the best use of their resources, that they knew what patients *really* needed, *really* wanted. They listened, and then they acted accordingly. ("So," Brian said to me at one point, with a big grin, "You want to buy some URLs?")

At WHA, they reenergized their focus on the experience and the relationship with a program called In Her Shoes, led by their chief medical officer. As in, "What would you want/do/need if you were in her shoes?" They highlighted moments when somebody was really taking the patient's perspective into account in staff meetings or clinical discussions. And as they continued to listen and to take that perspective, their practice evolved.

One thing they were hearing—again, not much of a surprise—was that patients wanted easier, more convenient access. And from Brian and the team's perspective, more convenient access might fill the void they saw in urgent care services. They began by adding evening and weekend hours, and then they addressed location and scheduling. Historically, ob-gyn practices have needed to be close to hospitals so that providers could pop over to the hospital to deliver a baby and then get back to the practice to see scheduled patients. If you're a woman, especially a woman who has had a baby, you've probably dealt with the inconveniences: long drives to wherever the closest hospital/medical office is. Canceled appointments when your doctor gets pulled into a delivery. Long waits for the doctor because a woman in labor doesn't deliver on schedule—babies are *just a nightmare* when it comes to sticking to schedules (how dare they!). Hospitals aren't necessarily close to where people work or live: a midday doctor's appointment that includes waiting for the doctor could eat two or three hours out of your schedule—which means it might be easier to just pop over to the closest "quick clinic" rather than go in to see a provider with whom you have an actual relationship.

WHA listened and then took the right action. They invested in more, smaller practices in satellite locations that would be convenient for their patients (close to work and home). They changed their operating model to have some providers staffing labor and delivery and some staffing the offices each day, which meant they weren't rescheduling patient visits because a doctor was suddenly called away to deliver a baby and reduced wait times for appointments. And the doctors could devote their attention to the patients at the hospital or at the office. The team found it liberating to be able to apply so much common sense to their strategic decisions.

I may have written the story above as a moment of revelation, but the truth is that WHA has always been concerned with relationship and access, and has made decisions and investments to support both. They were one of the few ob-gyn practices to offer full on-site lab services and some imaging services before these became common. Today they offer state-of-the-art mammography that you can schedule as part of your annual well woman's exam. In January, they opened a nurse-midwife birthing center for all of the patients who weren't interested in having a baby in a hospital. They can now offer the full range of care for pregnant women with different risk levels and different desires for birthing experiences, meaning the relationship between the practice and the patient remains intact, regardless. It's win-win all around.

Of course, each of these decisions has been carried out on a strong business platform, and each has made good financial sense in the long run. But other decisions, like an urgent care center, might have looked good, too, in a by-the-numbers sort of way. It's only the combination of the relationship, the science, and the financials that is making WHA as strong as it is in delivering great health care.

"As we've grown since 2011, it's been challenging," Brian said. "We cover the Portland metropolitan area, but Portland is different. We have a lot of different submarkets, with their own dynamics and their own needs. I might think, 'Hey, the Northwest Gynecology Center is a good solution for more sectors, so we should put one in this area or that area.' And then the feedback comes in that the patients don't really want that kind of practice or those services. It challenges me to really dial in and be more attuned to what people want.

"We're given just moments in time when we can enter into people's lives when they're vulnerable or frustrated," Brian adds. "What they're looking for is a connection and trust that we're going to do whatever we can for them, on a service level and a clinical level. To me, the art and science is really creating that trust and becoming a reliable partner in their health care."

✹

The story at the start of the section about the poorly located party only became more tragic, I'm afraid. As the husband toured around with his wife, he pointed proudly to the frozen Bellini maker he had rented. She loves Bellinis, but she hates frozen drinks. When she went to pour herself a glass of wine, she discovered that all that remained of her very favorite was a half bottle left over from dinner the night before. He had hired a band they had liked at a wedding they attended, but had given them a song list that didn't include most of her favorites. Unsurprisingly, a year later, they were divorced.

We've fallen into a similar pattern in health care over the last decades: We don't ask people what they really want, we certainly aren't listening to the answers when they do tell us, but we're definitely taking action—as if we're sure we know the best choice. But we don't. If we keep refusing to pay attention to what patients, providers, and practice staff tell us they want, we shouldn't be surprised when they divorce themselves, in one way or another, from the goals we all claim to aspire to—or even from health care entirely. We have a lot to learn from Brian and his team at Women's Healthcare Associates about how to listen, and then act accordingly.

The Right Approach
Ask the people the right questions, genuinely listen to the answers, and then take the right action.

The Right Question
How Can We Give the Right People Control?

Allow me to pull your attention back to the opening chapter of this book, the pages where I described the "business in the front, party in the back" reality of the symbol of the modern health-care experiences—the inappropriately revealing hospital gown.

Sure, you never feel confident and secure in one, but now imagine that you aren't the patient, your parent is. You're bringing your mom or dad to the hospital for a procedure that has you both feeling frightened and vulnerable. You're there to help, but when you get into the pre-op patient room, you aren't quite sure what to do. Your parent has to change into the gown, and there's nowhere for you to go, no curtain to draw, no way to be present without everybody feeling even more embarrassed. Do you turn and stare into the corner like the creepy guy at the end of *The Blair Witch Project*, or do you try to act nonchalant, even though it's been decades since you've seen your parent in anything less than a bathing suit? If your family has, in the last few generations, immigrated from a country where nudity is much less taboo—say, one of the Scandinavian countries, land of the family sauna—you're all set. But here in America, we tend to be so concerned about seeing other people's perfectly natural private parts that even a basic wardrobe malfunction can bring the country to a conversational standstill for a week after the Super Bowl. I tend to fall right in with that norm, I'm afraid.

So what's a kid supposed to do—leave and seem uncaring or unhelpful, or stay and cause humiliation all around?

This short, confounding moment in health care rose to the level of design challenge at Virginia Mason's Main Clinic in downtown Seattle. It came up because the team was redesigning a floor of their Lindeman Pavilion to create a new surgical suite from scratch. Along the way, they thought to ask patients an interesting question: "How would you like to experience this day?" But here's the more curious thing. This wasn't a survey or a focus group or an item on a pre-discharge questionnaire. They asked the question of patients who were actually a part of the design team, who were participating in the redesign and remodeling of the floor. Who else was on the team? Physicians, anesthesiologists, nurses, techs, janitors, administrative staff, accountants, architects—all there to look at the change from every facet and help support the care of the patient. As any good architect who has worked on a hospital redesign will tell you, the process doesn't begin with drawings, but with interviews with representatives of more than a hundred different constituencies who pass through a hospital each day. What they often find is that the needs of those different groups are sometimes diametrically opposed to one another: What a nurse needs might be the direct opposite of what a physician or X-ray technician needs. The art of architecture comes in part from meeting those different needs in a workable and elegant work space. It is a sensibility that Virginia Mason shares: At their clinic, change is in the hands of the people who either do the work or experience the work every day. And they put the needs of the patient at the forefront of everything they do.

What was their solution to this human problem that stemmed from human emotions? Would you believe small companion areas in the rooms where family or friends could be present without feeling in the way and without experiencing the full Monty? Simple, commonsense solution, no?

What I just described is one story Dr. Ryan Pong shared to describe the difference of Virginia Mason's approach to managing all aspects of their organization, what they call the Virginia Mason Production System. If it sounds like a manufacturing term, you're not wrong. It was adopted after leaders at Virginia Mason studied the Toyota system for high-quality, efficient, customer-driven car manufacturing and used it to improve their delivery of high-quality, efficient, patient-driven health care. These are the places where the master's in medical management part of me tends to geek out—I've been known to go weak in the knees for things like Six Sigma and lean management systems. So the business management piece of me wants to explain that by using the principles of rapid process improvement workshops, standard work, daily tours of the facilities by the leaders to look for unsolved challenges or problems, and more, Virginia Mason maximized their service delivery. However, the normal human woman part of me would rather just say: They came, they saw, they listened, they applied common sense, and then they did smart stuff.

If you meet somebody from Virginia Mason, don't bother making a joke about treating patients like cars coming off the assembly line. They've heard them all, and the jokes tend to die off when people see their data, their results, the patient satisfaction, their national rankings, and especially, the deep fulfillment and passion of the people who work there. Frankly, it's a little like talking to members of a cult. They tend to gush—and rightfully so. Just since early 2016, they've won national and regional awards for patient safety, for patient experience, for clinical excellence, for quality health care— even for being one of the "greenest" hospitals in America.

"How do we always keep our true north of putting the patient interests at the top of everything we do?" Dr. Pong, an anesthesiologist who came to Virginia Mason for his residency and never left, shared this question as the guiding light of their approach. "That means allowing the frontline staff to make decisions on how things should change, and to make the changes that will directly affect their work. As a physician, I find that really cool." Sarah Patterson, who is now the executive sensei but was the chief operating officer for nine years and one of the forces behind their revolution, shared the story of a primary care doctor who had worked at Virginia Mason and had left to work in a smaller private practice. She returned four or five years later, and when Sarah asked her why, she said that all of the organizations she looked at had the same problems, but at Virginia Mason, they had a method for solving them.

And here's where I might go all geeky again: What she was talking about was the team approach to continuous improvement that is the driving force behind how they tackle quality, safety, and even costs. Sarah explains it very simply: "I look at our jobs as leaders as supporting our staff in designing processes that help them do the right thing for patients, that deliver outstanding quality of care with the least amount of waste." A friend at another practice describes this kind of work in slightly earthier terms: Don't do dumb stuff, and don't make people do dumb stuff. If your people tell you that they're being asked to do dumb stuff, listen to them, get rid of the dumb stuff, and *let them design* smart stuff instead.

Before Virginia Mason started the journey they're on now, people sometimes felt conflicted between what they thought were competing priorities of cost control and quality. These are the foundations of today's so-called patient-centered care movement, and there's not a person working in health care today who doesn't relate to those conflicts on some level. "Our board challenged us with a question as we were putting together a new strategic plan," explained Gary Kaplan, CEO, in one of many articles about Virginia Mason's approach. " 'Who is your customer?' Like everyone in health care, we said the patient. But the board didn't accept that. We began to do a deep dive on our processes and came to realize that they were designed around us, the doctors, the nurses, the people working in the organization."[107] It's true. Patient-centric care is a great buzz phrase, but it often doesn't mean much because the systems and processes in health care tend to support those who pay for care and those providing the care, not those receiving the care. At Virginia Mason, they changed that.

Sounds good in principle. But does continuously improving to be more efficient really lend itself to never making a choice that sacrifices the patients' needs or safety? Turns out, yes, it does. In fact, Virginia Mason is proving that without a strict focus on high quality care, from the patient's perspective, it's almost impossible to reduce costs and waste through process because you aren't addressing the human problems that lead to inappropriate, ineffective care. And since everybody is involved in every change, senseless, purposeless, ineffective, soon-to-be-reversed change is kicked to the curb.

Take their primary care internal medicine practice, which was under a lot of pressure, especially from falling reimbursement rates, when they started down this path in 2002. In fact, the group hadn't been profitable in *thirty-four years*—more than three decades of negative income. Morale was not great because doctors felt so much pressure to see more patients that many were at the office until eight or nine o'clock at night finishing paperwork. The group was given extra resources to use the new change system to dramatically improve their practice—to improve the patient experience and reduce waste. They redesigned the flow of patients through the full process of admissions, nurse intakes, and doctor's exam. They redesigned the lab operations. They redesigned ... well, most things. And the results were astounding. For the first time in thirty-four years, the practice earned a profit. Far more important, though, they reduced the turnaround time for normal lab results from twenty-five days to just *two* days—imagine waiting twenty-five days to hear about lab results—and access improved because doctors were able to see more patients in a day. With improved workflows, those doctors were able to leave at six o'clock every night.[108]

They didn't stop there. They also targeted for improvement one of the great frustrations of health care these days: the endless "I call and miss you, you call and miss me, I call back and miss you again" game of epic phone tag. More than likely, at some point, you've been shunted into voice mail, waited hours or even days to hear back, then gotten a message to call the office, to which you responded with another message. It's exhausting. The team at Virginia Mason didn't like it either. It created frustration for everybody, and it was incredibly inefficient and wasteful. So they dramatically redesigned their call system. They focused on handling calls the first time in and handing patients over to live people. They prioritized calls for physicians so that they could easily return urgent messages throughout the day. Requests that couldn't be handled on the first call generally got a response or a call back within an hour. The result, of course, was that patients were happier and were better served with timely information, and the volume of calls (by cutting out all the callbacks) dropped dramatically, which saved the staff time and frustration. And so on and so on.[109]

Virginia Mason was able to get rid of the waiting room at their ambulatory care clinic by improving the flow of care. They made changes in how their nurses work in ways that increased the time they had in each shift to be with patients, soaring from 35 percent to 90 percent. They were also the first team in Washington State to offer a new, safer method for preventing stroke. They're on the leading edge of pancreatic cancer treatment.

Frankly, if you're sick or if you need to see a doctor, you might really want to consider Virginia Mason.

The number one reason, though, comes from another powerful statement from Dr. Pong. "The Virginia Mason Production System allows me to be a physician in the truest sense, where I really only have to worry about taking care of patients. It allows me to be a great physician. We are freed up to have that really meaningful connection with the patient." Somewhere Sir William Osler is smiling. It should also be said that Dr. Pong also spends time on regular improvements and efforts to drive efficiency, working in partnership with patients and everybody else to make the best kind of change happen, to create a virtuous cycle of caring. He has found that when you get control over the change, it feels empowering rather than debilitating. "You can't empower the patient without empowering the physician and care team first," he explained. That sound you hear is the collective sigh of a million physicians, raising their hands while offering an "Amen."

I am a firm believer in the idea that the people we desperately need in the process of innovation and care redesign are patients and providers, but in many organizations and certainly at the macro level, they're either being shut out or burnt out. Chris Trimble, a bestselling author on innovation and a professor at the Dartmouth Center for Health Care Delivery Science, captured perfectly one of the greatest problems of innovation in our system:

> I have received the strongest negative reactions to the notion of physicians doing the fixing from policy experts who hold a particular point of view on why the system is broken in the first place. That view, presented in the starkest possible terms, is as follows: Physicians have too much power. Furthermore, physician education inculcates a level of arrogance that leads to subtle abuse of that power. It encourages physicians to operate too much, prescribe too often,

and spend too carelessly. It invites physicians to design care not for patients but for their own convenience. It tempts physicians to view themselves as individual superheroes and their non-physicians' colleagues as diminutive minions. For those that hold this point of view, any effort to empower physicians, such as this book, is readily dismissed as pouring fuel on the fire.[110]

I absolutely agree, and I think it's great that Trimble is trying to encourage physicians to be a part of the innovation process (this passage comes from his book *How Physicians Can Fix Health Care*). However, until we remove some of the burdens they already face that sap their time, their energy, and their motivation, it isn't likely to happen. That is precisely what they have done at Virginia Mason: They have found a way to get out of the way of doctors doing their best and highest work in partnership with patients. The result is that everybody—from the janitor to the patient to the scheduler to the physician—has a willingness and an energy for owning the kind of positive change most health-care organizations need. Amen, indeed.

> **The Right Approach**
> Create the type of empowered partnerships
> that demand balance in the art, science,
> and business of medicine.

In 1902, Mary Anderson was riding on snowy New York streets and couldn't see through the windshield. She asked, "Why doesn't someone create a device to remove snow?" In 1970, Bernard Sadow was dragging two heavy suitcases through an airport. He asked, "Wouldn't this be easier if these things had wheels?" In 1996, Reed Hastings dreaded telling his wife that he had huge late fees on the movies he had rented. He wondered, "What if video rental businesses were run like health clubs, with a monthly fee?"

Like these inventors of the windshield wiper, the rolling suitcase, and Netflix, the organizations I've written about here have discovered the power that a well-focused question can have on driving change. Of course, these questions led to many more questions in each innovator's journey, to get to the source of truth in his or her industry. But people and organizations who are driven to make things better—in health care and elsewhere—seem to abide by a quote from artist Chuck Close: "Ask yourself an interesting enough question and your attempt to find a tailor-made solution to that question will push you to a place where, pretty soon, you'll find yourself all by your lonesome—which I think is a more interesting place to be." In some regards, these practices are all by their lonesome, and they're certainly in more interesting places.

We need answers to a lot of questions in health care today, but we also need a place to start. That's what the three questions in this chapter are designed to do—to create a foundation to begin a larger conversation. We know they work because we're seeing them in action. I encourage you to consider using them to help spark whatever change you are hoping to drive in your world today.

CHAPTER 9

Insisting on the Impossible

*Starting a new conversation in
health care begins with shifting away from
some of the old ones—and believing we can
put excellence, not mediocrity, at the
heart of medicine once again.*

O NE OF THE GREAT INNOVATIONS of the past hundred years started with a question from a three-year-old and an inventor willing to turn conventional wisdom on its head to begin a new conversation—an inventor who also happened to be one of Steve Jobs's heroes.

His name was Edwin Land. While vacationing with his family in Santa Fe, New Mexico, in 1943, Land was taking photographs of the rugged New Mexican landscape when he turned his attention to the young girl with the big personality standing next to him— his three-year-old daughter, Jennifer. She loved to have her photograph taken. What she didn't love was the two or three weeks it usually took to have the film turned into pictures before she could see them. Young Jennifer asked him an innocent question. Why did she have to *wait* to see the photo? Why couldn't she see it *now*?

Land wasn't just any other dad—he happened to be a brilliant chemist who had been obsessed with the interplay of light and polarity for nearly two decades, a brilliant chemist who had dropped out of Harvard (sound familiar?) to research and develop light-polarizing filters, eventually inventing a product for Eastman Kodak he had named the Polaroid.[111] He hadn't known how to build what Kodak wanted when he accepted the order, but as he explained later, "If you are able to state a problem—any problem—and it is important enough, then the problem can be solved."[112]

But his daughter's question was something different. As Warren Berger describes in his book *A More Beautiful Question*, seventy years before instant photography became a ubiquitous part of our twenty-first-century lives, Land took her question as a challenge, wondering, "Why *not* design a picture that can be developed right away?"[113]

The idea consumed him. Solving the question would require him to evolve some conventional truths that had long defined the industry. Traditional photography had always required a darkroom, but instant photography would necessitate the creation of a "darkroom" within the camera. Traditional photography required chemicals to be applied in sequence, while instant photography would need those chemicals to be applied *all at once*. Traditional photography required the creation of a *negative*; instant photography would involve the creation of a *positive*. The solution to his daughter's challenge would force something much bigger: a paradigm shift toward new ways of thinking to enable a profoundly different result.

Fortunately, as biographer Victor McElheny would recall, Land was a man who would "run through brick walls" if necessary.[114] Four years later, the Polaroid instant camera debuted during the holiday rush and completely sold out on the first day. Over the decades that followed, Polaroid sales increased a hundred times while the company became an American mainstay. It was adored by photographers from Ansel Adams to Andy Warhol to my dad, who used it to capture images of me during my awkward teen years that I have yet to purge from my brain.

Land himself would go on to hold more patents than any American before him except Thomas Edison. Years later, Jobs said of his hero, "Dr. Edwin Land was a troublemaker ... Not only was he one of the great inventors of our time but, more important, *he saw the intersection of art and science and business* and built an organization to reflect that."[115]

It is no accident that this chapter shares a title with McElheny's inspired biography of the man, because Edwin Land was a creative force who spent his life rejecting mediocrity and seeking better solutions while "insisting on the impossible." I share this story because I believe it's time for all of us who are frustrated with the current state of American health care to take a page from Land and rediscover our own passion for excellence, insist on the impossible again, and create a better path forward by bringing the art, science, and business of medicine back into balance.

In a world where American creativity has created breakthrough drugs, therapies, and treatments that have improved life for billions around the world, I don't think we have to accept that health care in the United States is just too complicated to see the broader benefit of those advancements here at home. I don't think we have to settle for accepting mediocrity in American medicine, making excuses for why the United States ranks so low in global health rankings despite spending more per citizen than any other nation on earth. I don't think we should resign ourselves to an entire generation of physicians feeling so burned out that they're retiring early just as a historic number of Americans are aging into their most health-care-intensive years. I don't think we have to accept that the most hopeful moment in the long history of medicine is also the most fraught moment in the modern history of American health care. I believe that we can replace incrementalism with innovation, complacency with creativity, mediocrity with miracles—and reach for excellence once again.

To quote the hero from the 1984 film *The Adventures of Buckaroo Banzai Across the 8th Dimension*, we should always remember that "no matter where you go, there you are." Translation: Part of the reason health care is stuck is because we keep waiting for a silver bullet, a savior to come along and make everything better. A 2012 study found that 82 percent of physicians believed they "had little ability to change the healthcare system" themselves.[116] But no matter where *we* go in American medicine, there *we* are. There isn't a savior waiting around the corner, just as there isn't a bogeyman who created the challenges described in the first seven chapters of this book. In reality, it's *us*—it has always been just us. And that, as we saw in chapter 8, is more than enough. If we are able to identify a need, any need, and it is important enough, then it can be solved.

In the last chapter, we saw how some of the leading medical practices in America are bringing the art, science, and business of medicine back into balance. They use their single source of truth—people—to drive their transformation, and ask the right fundamental questions about those people to produce better outcomes at lower costs with greater satisfaction. Just as those questions provide a starting point for shifting the art, science, and business of medicine back to balance to make health care sustainable, there are fundamental paradigm shifts away from old ways of thinking and toward the new that we need at the macro level in order to encourage the profoundly unique solutions necessary in health care today. I believe these paradigm shifts are the starting point for initiating a new conversation about how we can move American health care past the mediocrity we are settling for today to reach for—and achieve—excellence once again.

In *The Shawshank Redemption*, which is my favorite movie, there is a scene in which Tim Robbins's character, Andy Dufresne, tells Morgan Freeman's character, Ellis Boyd "Red" Redding, about his yearning to get out of jail and run off to Mexico to begin a new life. Red tells Andy, who is serving a life sentence, that it's not healthy for him to dream of escaping. Andy says, "I guess it comes down to a simple choice: get busy living or get busy dying." We've been busy dying: we've seen where the current health care road will take us.

It's time we get busy living—starting with these five shifts.

Five Paradigm Shifts to Get Back to Balance

1. From **money** as an incentive to **time** as an incentive
2. From more **complexity** to more **simplicity**
3. From more **metrics** to more **relationships**
4. From **process-driven** to **outcome-driven**
5. From **zero-sum** ("I win, you lose") to **non-zero-sum** ("we all win")

SHIFT ONE
From Money as an Incentive to Time as an Incentive

As a young doctor practicing medicine in New York City, Danielle Ofri had read too many stories about patients who felt like their doctors didn't listen to them. She worried that she might be turning into one of those physicians, admitting to herself that she often felt so overwhelmed with the number of important decisions she had to juggle on behalf of her patients during each office visit that a single question could throw her off her game.

One day she decided to conduct an experiment, to see how many details a primary care doctor like her juggled in the course of a typical twenty-minute office visit. For one patient, a fifty-six-year-old woman with multiple chronic conditions—including obesity, diabetes, hypertension, and high cholesterol—she recorded all of her thoughts. As she later shared in *The Lancet*, immediately after walking into the exam room, her inner dialogue began:

> Good thing she did her blood tests. Glucose is a little better. Cholesterol isn't great. May need to think about starting a statin. Are her liver enzymes normal?
>
> Her weight is a little up. I need to give her my talk about five fruits and vegetables and 30 min of walking each day.
>
> Diabetes: how do her morning sugars compare to her evening sugars? Has she spoken with the nutritionist lately? Has she been to the eye doctor? The podiatrist?
>
> Her blood pressure is good but not great. Should I add another

BP med? Will more pills be confusing? Does the benefit of possible better blood pressure control outweigh the risk of her possibly not taking all of her meds?

Her bones are a little thin on the DEXA. Should I start a bisphosphonate that might prevent osteoporosis? But now I'm piling yet another pill onto her, and one that requires detailed instructions. Maybe leave this until next time?

How are things at home? Is she experiencing just the usual stress of life, or might there be depression or anxiety disorder lurking? Is there time for the depression questionnaire?

Health maintenance: when was her last mammogram? PAP smear? Has she had a colonoscopy since she turned 50? Has she had a tetanus booster in the past 10 years? Does she qualify for a pneumonia vaccine?[117]

As the young doctor conducts this inner monologue, the patient interrupts to say that her back has been aching for the past few months, which makes Ofri—who is "juggling so many thoughts" that she "needs to resolve before the clock winds down"—feel like holding her hand up to stop the patient from talking. It's only then that we realize that the entire visit to this point has taken place silently, with Ofri looking at the computer screen and typing in an electronic health record while the patient sits behind her. What she worries may be the straw that breaks the camel's back comes when the patient pulls a form out of her bag and insists that it be completed by Friday or she may lose her coverage. Ofri responds that she must conduct a physical exam first, where she "barrels though the basics" before investigating the back pain. Inputting all the information into the computer—again, silently—she realizes the appointment has run past its allotted time. Hitting "print," she hands the patient her prescriptions and begins to make her way to the door, only to hear the patient ask about her insurance form, which Ofri admits to having completely forgotten about.

This is just one of ten nearly identical patient visits she conducts in the course of the afternoon. She later calculates that the fifty-six-year-old woman had seven medical issues, which led to 35 separate thoughts; for all ten patients, she calculated about 350 thoughts. She also supervised five residents that morning at the academic medical center where she worked, each of which saw four patients, generating 10 thoughts each—or 200 total, which Ofri was also responsible for. All told, she juggled 550 thoughts in the course of one day.

There are certainly other professionals that juggle just as many if not more thoughts in the course of the day—teachers juggle more than 2,000—but as Ofri argues, "if I do a good job juggling 98 percent of the time, that still leaves 10 thoughts that might get lost in the process," any one of which could turn into a disaster for which she could get sued. The next day, she will do it all over again.

It's never been easy to practice medicine. But Ofri's story proves that as we transition as an industry from treating acute conditions (where you have a pain or illness that gets healed) to one managing chronic conditions (where drugs and therapies help you live for decades with illnesses that used to cause early deaths, like heart disease or high blood pressure), the number of drugs and treatments available to help manage that care puts an intense pressure on doctors to juggle an ever-growing list of options and responsibilities. As 75 million baby boomers move into retirement, those pressures will be exacerbated in ways that will continue to crowd out the time that the art of medicine needs to thrive.

As we've seen, the stimulant used to encourage "good physician behavior" today is money, in the form of incentives intended to ensure that boxes are checked or penalties when they are not. We shouldn't be opposed to incentives that reduce waste or achieve lower costs, but only if those things are done with the patient's welfare in mind first and foremost—meaning only if the time needed to carry out the art and science of medicine is factored in. We don't need to be told that fewer than one in seven doctors today feel they have the time to achieve what they want to achieve in their day. Ofri's story is all we need to understand why. Once again, it comes back to the simple reality that for health-care providers, medical practices, and their patients, time is the most valuable commodity. Rather than starting with the question "How do we use money to reward good behavior?" we should insist that payers and lawmakers ask instead, "How do we use time to encourage good outcomes?" It's time we give our practitioners the time they need to establish the trusting relationships and deliver the care necessary to achieve the outcomes we all desire.

SHIFT TWO
From More Complexity to More Simplicity

When I think about the incredible opportunities that exist within health care to create a path forward rooted in excellence instead of mediocrity, one number always comes to mind: 15,948. In 1997, it might have seemed like a completely normal number. In 2017, 15,948 borders on the absurd.

Believe it or not, in the year 2016, 15,948 is the number of faxed pages Jonathan Bush, cofounder and CEO of the electronic health records provider athenahealth, estimated the average physician handled each year.[118] That's an average of 307 pages each week, or roughly 44 pages a day. Even if you use just half of the active physicians in the United States to account for overlap in sending and receiving, doctors send enough faxes back and forth to circle the earth roughly 47 times in a year.

I routinely meet millennials who have never seen or used a fax machine. Yet in an era when everyone else has moved on to the digital transmission of information, doctors' offices still party like it's 1997—the year that sales of fax machines in the United States peaked[119]—because of the complexity set in motion by one law. As *PC World* explained in 2014, "Thanks to the HIPAA (Health Insurance Portability and Accountability Act), documents transmitted between various doctors, labs, and insurers have to be 'secure.'" The language of HIPAA is about as clear as fifty miles of muddy water, but it requires only that doctors engage in "reasonable safeguards" to protect patient privacy when sending messages, regardless of the medium. Over time, this has been interpreted by most doctors to mean that faxes are okay, but email isn't—because email can be hacked. (Never mind that fax machines usually sit in the open, or that e-faxes *can* be hacked.)

In other words, at the end of a decade in which the United States has invested $30 billion to encourage medical practices to improve communication by moving to electronic health records, since EHRs are still interoperable, the primary mode of exchanging sensitive medical information today is the same technology that reached its peak when Cabbage Patch Kids and parachute pants were still a *thing*. One study found that HIPAA rules and outdated technology cost hospitals alone $8.3 billion a year while increasing the average discharge time for patients by 50 percent.[120]

Like the store manager in the movie *Clerks* who is forced to work on his day off and complains throughout the whole film, "I'm not even supposed to be here today," this isn't even what HIPAA was supposed to do when it was passed in 1996. It was designed to allow employees to move health insurance from job to job while using technology to make health care more *efficient*. But like so many other well-intentioned health-care laws and regulations that we've discussed in this book, it morphed over time into something much bigger. And like sexually transmitted diseases, none of them ever go away. Layers simply keep getting added on, year after year. The laws and regulations governing Medicare alone, which ran for fewer that 1,000 pages when it was first passed in 1965, now run for more than 130,000 pages—all of which are active and in force.[121] And since federal, state, and local regulators, along with private insurance companies, don't check with one another before adding new layers, it just keeps snowballing—making health care second only to nuclear energy as the most complex and regulated industry in America.

As Edwin Land and Steve Jobs and any of the leaders we profiled in chapter 8 would tell us, the answer to improving a complex industry is not to propose solutions that just add more complexity. It is to *simplify*. What if, like the requirement that Congress cut a dollar of spending for every dollar added, health regulators agreed that for every new responsibility they want to require of patients, physicians, or medical practices, they first take one away? What would happen if we defined a national standard that at least 75 percent of the time of a physician had to be reserved for direct patient care—not on billing or EHRs or checking boxes? What if, by the year 2020, all EHRs in America were required to speak the same language and fluidly talk with one another? What if we could simplify billing to require only a single form, no matter where you went?

It's not like other industries haven't been here. Banking has figured out how to seamlessly move money and information from one institution to another, in different states, in different countries, across continental borders. The technology industry has figured out how to create application program interfaces (APIs) that allow developers from around the world to produce apps that work with platforms like Mac or PC or Android. The aviation industry, the energy industry—the list of those industries that have worked hard to simplify in the face of complexity to improve experience and safety goes on and on and on, while in health care the reverse is happening.

It's the difference between accepting mediocrity and aiming for excellence. It's time we replace complexity with simplicity to bring balance back to the art, science, and business of medicine to achieve excellence once again.

SHIFT THREE
From More Metrics to More Relationships

I loved the actress Mindy Kaling when she played a gossipy office worker in the American version of the TV show *The Office*. I love her even more as the star of her own show, *The Mindy Proj-*

ect, in which she plays a talented but awkward obstetrician with a nutty romantic history who is more than occasionally overmatched by life.

In one episode from the show's first season, a charming and handsome ob-gyn in her practice has to deliver bad news to a pregnant woman whose obesity poses a risk to her child. But the doctor is such a saint in the eyes of the woman and her husband that he can't bring himself to deliver the news. When he asks Mindy to do it for him, she reluctantly agrees and then proceeds to tell the woman, painfully, that she needs to lose weight. Angry, the woman tells Kaling that "she's no Keira Knightley" herself, prompting a defensive Kaling to shout back that she fluctuates "between chubby and curvy." The scene ends with the husband accepting that both he and his wife need to lose weight—and with the couple hating Kaling.

I was amused a short time later to see this scene included in a *New Yorker* story by Lisa Rosenbaum about the new era of "patient satisfaction" we are living in today.[122] As I first mentioned in the opening chapter, in 2012, the federal government announced that any hospital that accepted Medicare would be required to have patients who received care fill out a twenty-seven-category patient satisfaction survey that scored everything from cleanliness to communication to pain management. Depending on those scores, hospitals could gain or lose an additional 2 percent of their reimbursement dollars—millions, for some. With Americans increasingly responsible for paying a larger share of their health-care costs, the movement to treat patients more like customers is not, on its face, a bad thing. But by now we now know two things: There is a big difference between intent and results in health-care policy, and tracking metrics doesn't necessarily help providers build the trust necessary to create the strong relationships that lie at the heart of better outcomes.

If the pregnant woman and her husband being "treated" by Mindy were asked to fill out a survey of the care they received, who do you think would come out with higher scores: the beloved doctor who refused to tell them bad news or the hapless doctor who incurred their wrath? This isn't a hypothetical question—not only are hospitals being rewarded or penalized based on satisfaction surveys, but an increasing number of physicians now have their pay and bonuses tied directly to their patient scores—because practices of a certain size that accept Medicare are now also required to use a similar survey or face a penalty. A growing body of anecdotal evidence shows that more and more, physicians are avoiding difficult conversations with patients for fear of having their pay diminished by bad scores. And it's a valid fear: Rosenbaum shared the results of a study that found that 69 percent of patients with terminal lung cancer and 81 percent of patients with terminal colon cancer didn't understand that chemotherapy wouldn't cure their disease—but the more their grim condition was explained to them, the less they liked the doctors who delivered the news.[123]

More troublingly, a study described in *The Atlantic* in 2015 found that two-thirds of the hospitals that performed worse than the national average in patient outcomes—hospitals "where a higher number of patients will die, be unexpectedly readmitted to the hospital, or suffer serious complications"—scored higher than the national average on patient satisfaction scores.[124] An article entitled "Patient Satisfaction Is Overrated" made waves in 2013 when it suggested that for many physicians, "The mandate is simple: Never deny a request for an antibiotic, an opioid pain medication, a scan, or an admission," citing one emergency room with bad ratings that even began to offer discharged patients "goody bags" of hydrocodone painkillers to increase their scores.[125] The evidence was troubling enough that Medicare announced in early 2017 that it was removing "pain management" as a category from the twenty-seven-point satisfaction survey.

I've argued that the good data that *effective* metrics provide are essential to advancing the science at the heart of evidence-based medicine. But I've also argued that not all metrics or standards are created equal, and we should not equate metric-tracking with trust-building, because to do so misses a crucial point: What looks good on paper and what drives the best outcomes in practice can be two very different things. Too often, what looks good on paper is what is possible to measure, not necessarily what is actually the best approach to caring for patients. And when we consider the costs of abiding by and tracking and reporting all of these metrics—the four hours of physician time, the eight hours of care team time, the $8 billion we spend as a nation every year—it's pretty clear that we're interfering with those best, relationship-building approaches.

Instead of spending so much more of our national time, resources, and attention in medicine on creating artificial metrics designed to incentivize good physician and provider behavior while unwittingly reinforcing bad behavior, let's give the art of medicine the room it needs to build trusting relationships in the way that the best doctors and medical practices have always done so: honestly, naturally, compassionately, and with the best outcomes for the patient squarely in mind.

SHIFT FOUR
From Process-Driven to Outcome-Driven

You may remember the secretly recorded 1971 Oval Office conversation between chief of staff John Ehrlichman and President Richard Nixon about the Kaiser Permanente approach to managing costs that was talked about in chapter 4. That discussion occurred at the very start of the current era of health care, an era that has seen process be consistently prioritized over outcomes. The thinking was originally sound: Process helps drive outcomes (and costs). But an obsession with process (and costs) as a way to gain control amid all of the variability in health care has distracted us, decade by decade, from the ultimate goal. It's classic trees instead of forest.

As it happens, one of the institutions today that has been working to bring the focus of health care and health professionals back from an emphasis on doing a defined set of *things* (process) to doing the right things that *drive the right results* (outcomes) is Kaiser Permanente.

If you've ever spent more than a few hours as a patient in a hospital, like one in Kaiser's now-nationwide system, you understand that patients are more dependent on nurses than on any other provider. Nurses are the ever-present caregivers who help patients with their needs from moment to moment, who are the push of a button away, and who are often the link with the hospital doctor or the specialist in charge of the patient's treatment. When nurses become essentially unavailable for forty-five minutes, it's a problem. At Kaiser, it happened with every shift change: Patients felt abandoned while the nurses disappeared to update the incoming staff. More than half an hour later, a new face would appear in the room, often missing details the patients felt were important.

Kaiser Permanente teamed up with IDEO, the icon of human-centered design, to improve the nurses' shift change.[126] What they realized together was that Kaiser had done a terrific job creating a process that worked well for their *nursing staff*—handoffs were clean, histories were covered. But that process paid little attention to the impact it had on the patients the medical personnel were all there to care for.

The IDEO team led groups of nurses through the systems design process, and the result was the Nurse Knowledge Exchange. Now shift changes happen at the patient's bedside and patients are encouraged to participate so that everybody feels comfortable with the information being passed on. Whiteboards in patient rooms contain personal details about the patient—family, pets, likes and dislikes. Shift changes happen quickly, efficiently, and patients and nurses are both more satisfied. There was a bit of revamping of the technology (the EHR) to help consolidate nurses' notes into a single simple screen, but the majority of the shift happened when the nurses considered their needs and experiences alongside those of the patient and found a way to improve both—because well-cared-for patients with reduced anxiety levels heal better and faster, and that's the right outcome.

As we've explored in chapters 2 and 8, we aren't asking the right questions in medicine anymore—*and* we're not achieving the right outcomes. Instead of asking, "How do we apply more science and business to develop the best processes?" we need to ask ourselves, "How do we get to what we really want: happier patients, lower cost, and better quality medicine? What is missing from the current picture that is preventing us from achieving what we want to achieve?"

Putting the emphasis on process too far separated from the outcomes it's supposed to be helping us achieve eats resources such as time and energy and money and adds to the complexity, as overlapping processes create confusion and conflict. We keep honing individual processes—as the efficiency-driven business side of medicine encourages us to do—rather than stepping away from the solutions directly in front of us and collaborating to create new, more excellent solutions that drive excellent outcomes.

If we are going to achieve the results we all want from America's health-care industry, we can't design the future of medicine with the first consideration being for an ever more efficient process, defined by formulas like billable hours divided by patients seen. We've got to begin with the outcomes we want—with a focus on the patient's welfare first and foremost, and with consideration for the art it takes to achieve the best results for the patient, just as Virginia Mason has done. Then we can reverse-engineer the process to achieve those results. With that approach, we'll achieve true, meaningful efficiency: the best outcomes with the least waste of energy, time, and money.

SHIFT FIVE
From Zero-Sum ("I Win; You Lose") to
Non-Zero-Sum ("We All Win")

On January 18, 2012, the Internet went dark. Threatened with the passage of two divisive copyright bills that many believed would lead to online censorship and would undermine Internet freedoms, thousands of websites—including Wikipedia, Google, Reddit, and Flickr—placed black banners over their logos and went dark for a full day. Visitors who clicked were directed to a page with information on the two bills and instructions on how to contact their elected officials.

By the end of the day, more than 10 million people had signed an online petition. Eight million people had visited the websites of their congressional representatives, causing them to crash. More than 100,000 phone calls flooded the U.S. Capitol. Three million emails and one million messages were sent to members of Congress.

Within forty-eight hours, both bills were pulled from consideration, never to be raised again. It was one of the most forceful displays of power in the Information Age, a startling reminder of the central role that online companies play in our increasingly digital economy.

For every frustrated or burned-out physician in America today, it would be understandable if they occasionally wondered about doing the same thing. After all, as we've seen, more than 80 percent of every action in medicine happens because a physician orders it. Just imagine, the thinking goes, if every single one of America's roughly 850,000 physicians stayed home for a day. Imagine if every surgeon, pediatrician, emergency room physician, and primary care doctor acted like the mom in that television commercial, who walks into a room and says, "I'm sorry, I have to call in sick today"—only to have the camera pivot to reveal that she is talking to her toddler. (Like that mom, it's absurd to consider doctors "going dark" for a million reasons, mainly because physicians—most of whom go into medicine because they are called to heal, save, or improve the lives of their fellow human beings—would never do that.) If physicians walked out, our health-care system—the practice of medicine—would come to a standstill.

But let's consider the idea on a bigger scale. The same thing would happen if nurses stopped caring for patients for a day, or medical practice managers stopped coordinating with patients or moving the information necessary to keep the system operating. The same thing would happen if the business side of medicine—the insurance companies and Medicare regulators—stopped paying the bills. The same thing would happen if the science side of medicine— the researchers in labs who run the tests and the scientists working to find the next generation of cures—stopped the greatest break-throughs in medical ingenuity from saving and improving lives.

As has probably become clear by this point in the book, I'm just as much a fan of movies as I am of medicine. I've always been one of those people who sit through the credits at the end of a movie, long before the geniuses who work on animated films and super-hero movies made it a requirement by adding an extra scene after the credits run. I'm always amazed by the number of names that scroll by, the literally thousands of people it takes—working on jobs big and small—to bring a movie from an idea to the screen. I think that one of the reasons that Michael Crichton was able to move so effortlessly from practicing medicine to eventually directing mov-ies, aside from the obvious fact of his brilliance, is that medicine is very much like the movies.

We may believe that it's a zero-sum game: That on everything from paying medical claims to regulating medical practices, for one side to win, somebody else needs to lose. But this is not true, and it's never been true. Health care has always been a nonzero practice, in a word made popular by the author Robert Wright: It's an industry in which each side should be able to win together, and in fact *can only win together*, at least on the things that truly matter. If we start by asking the right questions, if we are able to shift some of the para-digms in thinking that are holding us back today, there is no reason why we can't begin a new conversation that truly moves American health care in a new direction—one that puts the needs of people at the center of the industry again, that reaches beyond mediocrity to excellence, and brings the art, science, and business of medicine back into balance to create a path forward for all of us that is sustainable.

As Edwin Land once said in a speech to his employees on why he insisted on the impossible and how he made it happen, "If you dream of something worth doing and then simply go to work on it … if you just think of, detail by detail, what you have to do next, it is a wonderful dream even though the end is a long way off, for there are about five thousand steps to be taken before we realize it; and start taking the first ten, and stay making twenty after, it is amazing how quickly you get through those five thousand steps."[127]

I guess it comes down to a simple choice: Get busy living or get busy dying. I vote that we get busy living. That's what back to balance means to me.

The Triad of Caduceus:
A New Way of Seeing the Symbol of Medicine

Walk into just about any medical practice, hospital, or pharmacy in America, and you'll see a familiar sight: a short golden rod entwined by two snakes and topped by a pair of wings. It's the popular symbol we've come to associate with American medicine.

Except that it has nothing to do with healing—or at least it didn't for 2,400 years.

As it turns out, there isn't one medical symbol associated with snakes, there are two: the one that everyone in America knows, and then the one that is actually associated with healing, or more specifically, the Greek god of healing and medicine, Asclepius. Asclepius was the son of Apollo and a human woman named Coronis. After Apollo had Coronis burned on a funeral pyre for falling in love with another human while pregnant with Asclepius (first removing the babe in what has been called history's first, and tensest, cesarean section), he entrusted Asclepius's upbringing to a centaur named Chiron, who was wise in the ways of the healing arts. Under the tutelage of the half man, half horse, Asclepius became a gifted physician.[128] One day while treating a patient, Asclepius was surprised by a snake and killed it with his staff—which was bad luck, since snakes were revered for their powers of healing and rejuvenation. The physician was amazed when another snake came along, fed herbs to the first snake, and brought it back to life. With this insight, Asclepius then used these same herbs to bring a man back to life.

From that day forward, Asclepius chose as his symbol a knotty tree limb entwined with a single serpent (and no wings), known as the rod of Asclepius. For the 2,400 years that followed, the rod of Asclepius served as the symbol of healing for physicians across the world. But a funny thing happened as America entered the twentieth century: The other symbol, the one we all know, the rod with the two snakes and wings, began to make inroads into the medical community.

It was the caduceus, or magic wand, of Hermes, the son of Zeus. He was the Greek god of merchants and thieves, the messenger between deities and mortals, the deliverer of information, the muse of eloquence, the inventor of magical incantations, and the force responsible for shepherding the dead into the underworld. His only connection to medicine was that, like modern physicians, he seemed to have too many responsibilities and not enough time in the day to accomplish them all well.

Hermes also had a mythical encounter with snakes. Happening upon two powerful serpents engaged in combat one day, the deity ended the battle by separating them with his wand, at which point the two snakes coiled around one another and fused on the wand. Hence the caduceus of Hermes was born. In the centuries that followed, his brand remained medicine-free. In fact, Hermes's only connection to anything approximating healing was to alchemists, who were revered for their mystical belief in the magical transformation of matter for many things, including healing.

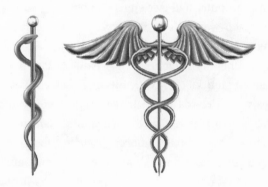

So, how did the caduceus become associated with medicine? By mistake.

According to Dr. Walter Friedlander, author of a lovingly authoritative book on the subject, the mix-up came in the nineteenth century, when a London publisher of medical books named John Churchill began to include the caduceus as a printer's mark on textbooks he exported to America. Some U.S. publishers followed suit, and it soon caught the eye of several physicians. The forerunner of the U.S. Public Health Service was one of the first to include the caduceus in its seal. Many others followed.[129]

By 1990, Friedlander found that 39 percent of professional medical associations and 76 percent of commercial organizations used the caduceus as the symbol of healing.[130] By 2014, the takeover was complete: A study of 200 doctors and 100 medical students found that 94 percent were completely unaware that the rod of Asclepius was the true symbol of healing—or even knew the story of the god of medicine at all.[131]

So yes, it's true: The nearly universal emblem of American health care today is a symbol long associated with the occult that never had anything to do with healing and actually signifies the movement of dead souls into the underworld. As a physician who has had that symbol as a constant part of my life for thirty years—heck, my husband nearly got it tattooed onto his ankle in a moment of youthful indiscretion while we were in medical school—that's just not good enough.

Here's my modest proposal: If the caduceus of Hermes is going to guide us going forward, it might be useful to think about it in a new way. Let's call it the triad of caduceus. I choose to see the golden rod—the foundation of the symbol—as the science of medicine; the snake that coils to the left as the art of medicine; and the snake that coils to the right as the business of medicine. It represents both the aspiration and the ideal of medicine, all three in balance—the art, science, and business of medicine—ready to help those wings take flight.

It can also serve as a constant reminder that there is no divine entity, no great savior, no outside force that's going to come along and make health care in America work as well in practice as in promise. I'll repeat, it's just *us*. It's always been just us—the same ones who discovered antibiotics, transplanted a human heart, sequenced the human genome, and nearly doubled the average life expectancy of every man and woman in America. The same ones who are beginning to turn the tide on diseases that have plagued humanity from the very beginning—who have also, it should be said, made do with a thin and drafty cotton gown for more than a century. *We* are the ones that we have been waiting for. And I believe with every ounce of my being: That's more than enough.

ACKNOWLEDGMENTS

The conventional wisdom is that it's not the destination, it's the journey. I would argue that in the case of this book, it's the people I met and worked with along the way. Completing this book took an entire tribe of people, and it's time to thank them.

I dedicated this book to practice leaders, and there are some very special practice leaders without whom this project wouldn't have been possible. I thank all three of the board chairs of MGMA-ACMPE who supported me through this project, including Ron Holder, who asked the big questions; Mickey Smith, who asked the tough questions; and Deb Wiggs, whose enthusiasm was infectious; as well as the entire board from 2015 to 2017, including Jim Barrett, Michael Biselli, Eric Crockett, Yvette Doran, Brad Esbaugh, Todd Grages, Bill Hambsh, Anne Hill, David Kelch, Kyle Mathews, Karen Marcelo, Rich Schlossberg, Amanda Smith, Jeff Smith, Marie Walton, and Shirley Zwinggi. Their feedback, stories, and insightful comments made this book so much better—and helped me to avoid pitfalls.

There are several other people who touched the book deeply and added to its unique voice: Victoria Hanley, a gifted and award-winning author in her own right, who offered me help and then actually gave it. You are a remarkable woman. Todd Evenson, thank you for your unrelenting faith, cheerleading, warmth, laughter, and steadfast insistence that my voice be heard through the book.

The executive team at MGMA—including Anders Gilberg, Tina Hogeman, Andrew Swanson, Shelly Waggoner, and Tracy Watrous—is such an amazing team, and I am so proud! Your commitment to transform health care for everyone is the engine that drives what we do every day. It's a privilege to work with each of you, and in some cases, occasionally, *for* you. You are such remarkable people, and it's the highlight of my career to have the privilege to work with you.

I give my heartfelt appreciation to my MGMA staff. Their commitment to our membership positively impacts medical practice every day.

Those people who were kind enough to consent to be interviewed —Rushika Fernandopulle, Brian Kelly, Dr. Ryan Pong, and Sarah Patterson—added their depth and substance to our project. These people are my personal heroes and have my profound gratitude.

In a previous book I thanked Mark Rumans, and here I do it again, for a different reason this time. He is a role model for physician leadership, and for the past decade or so he has been a great friend, the source of endless moral support, and a damn good sounding board. Most important, he is a person who doesn't judge me, who encourages me, and who has the courage to "speak truth" to redheads.

I would be remiss and a stereotypical ungrateful first child if I didn't thank my parents again. They gave me life, supported me through the tough times and the good times and the crazy times (even when they were completely dubious about where it was all going), and have gifted me with such great material to write about!

Ellen Boyd, thank you again for making this all possible. Which reminds me, thank-yous go to three people: Carole Peet, who taught me about leadership; Phil Harkins, who taught me about discipline; and Sheri Jacobs, who taught me about authentic professional passion. Also, a special thanks to Russell Owens, who taught me about being a warrior with soft eyes and having an iron will wrapped in cotton ... or not. All of these people taught me so much of what was necessary for this book.

This project started with good intentions on a bright warm Colorado spring day with brilliant blue skies, and then "got real" twenty-four hours and three bottles of wine later in the midst of a freak blizzard that closed the airports. It was over dinner at my house that I got to really know my editorial panel as magnificent people, and they are fabulous companions for this journey. (And no, I don't mean *have been* here, as this journey may never end!) They are all brilliant, funny, and totally committed ... and you can interpret that any way you wish, Lari Bishop, Kris Pauls, and Paul Orzulak.

Dear Lari, you are simultaneously my sage and my spiritual counselor. When I met you for the first time, I thought it was just for this project, and now I hope this is just the first of many projects for us. You are such a wise soul—and I regret that you have enriched me far more than I you. Thank you. Kris, you are the most remarkable publisher I've ever met. You're infinitely patient, kind, and mostly tactful, and you listen incredibly well—you're the glue, and even better, you're a trusted friend. I wish you laughter, joy, and deep mystery for your next adventure—mazel tov! Finally, to the person I am the most grateful for: Paul. Dear Paul, and I mean this from the bottom of my heart, your spirit is what makes this project so special. This book would not be what it is without you, and that is the very highest compliment I know how to give.

Last, but certainly not least, thanks to my husband Michael, who listened to hundreds of hours of me talking about the ideas in the book. This book wouldn't be here without you. You are a remarkable man, partner, coconspirator, and consigliere, and when necessary, you serve as the painful voice of reason. Every night I consider myself so blessed that you are in my life. I hope I can someday be the person I see reflected in your eyes.

Much love to everyone,
Halee

SOURCE NOTES

CHAPTER 1

The passage from the article "In America, the Art of Doctoring is Dying" by Jerald Winakur (February 12, 2016) is reprinted by permission of the author.

CHAPTER 3

The story of "Meagan" originally appeared in *The Life You Save* by Patrick Malone (Da Capo, 2009): 30–34 and appears by permission of the publisher.

CHAPTER 4

The story of "Gloria Brown" and BioPlus Specialty Pharmacy appears in the forthcoming book *Predictable Results* by Patrick Thean (Leadline, Inc., 2017) and appears by permission of the author.

CHAPTER 5

Material from the article "The Story of a Man Who Was a Very Good Cook" by Mark Williams (2016) was originally published at KevinMD.com and appears by permission of the author.

CHAPTER 6

The passage from "The EHR Interface and My Personal Moment of Zen" by Margalit Gur-Arie (December 2, 2012) was originally published at KevinMD.com and is reprinted by permission of the author.

Passages from "Clinical Education and the Electronic Health Record: The Flipped Patient" by Jeffrey Chi and Abraham Verghese (December 10, 2014): 2331–2332 are reprinted by permission of the *Journal of The American Medical Association*.

The passage and stories from *Touching Strangers* by Richard Renaldi (Aperture Foundation, 2014) are reprinted by permission of the publisher.

SOURCE NOTES

CHAPTER 7

The passage from "A Physician's Open Letter to Medicare Patients" by Rebekah Bernard (November 1, 2015) was originally published at KevinMD.com and is reprinted by permission of the author.

CHAPTER 9

The passage from "Neuron Overload and the Juggling Physician" by Danielle Ofri (November 27, 2010) is reprinted by permission of *The Lancet*. Copyright © 2010. Published by Elsevier Ltd. All rights reserved.

REFERENCES

1. White, Jess, "Are New Hospital Gowns the Key to Patient Satisfaction?" *Healthcare Business & Technology*, April 6, 2015, available at healthcarebusinesstech.com/hospital-gown-update/.

2. Luthra, Shefali, "Despised Hospital Gowns Get Fashion Makeovers," CNN.com, April 1, 2015, available at cnn.com/2015/04/01/health/hospital-gown -fashion-makeover/.

3. Gholipour, Bahar, "Keep Your Pants, and Your Dignity, at the Hospital," *Live Science*, September 22, 2014, available at livescience.com/47947-hospital -patients-should-wear-own-cloths.html.

4. Luthra, Shefali, "Hospital Gowns Get a Makeover," *The Atlantic*, April 4 2015, available at theatlantic.com/health/archive/2015/04/hospital-gowns-get -a-makeover/389258/.

5. Ofri, Danielle, "The Art of Medicine: Neuron Overload and the Juggling Physician," *The Lancet*, vol. 376 (November 2010): 1820–1821, available at thelancet.com/pdfs/journals/lancet/PIIS0140-6736(10)62157-5.pdf.

6. "Allocation of Physician Time in Ambulatory Practice: A Time and Motion Study in 4 Specialties," *Annals of Internal Medicine*, December 6, 2016, available at annals.org/aim/article/2546704/allocation-physician-time -ambulatory-practice-time-motion-study-4-specialties.

7. "Doctors-in-Training Spend Very Little Time at Patient Bedside, Study Finds," Johns Hopkins Medicine New Release, April 23, 2013, available at hopkinsmedicine.org/news/media/releases/doctors_in_training_spend_very _little_time_at_patient_bedside_study_finds.

8. Winakur, Jerald, "In America, the Art of Doctoring Is Dying," *The Washington Post*, February 12, 2016, available at washingtonpost.com /opinions/the-dying-art-of-doctoring/2016/02/12/bb08a16a-cddo-11e5-88cd -753e80cd29ad_story.html?utm_term=.555b5438a2a7.

9. The Physicians Foundation, "2014 Survey of America's Physicians: Practice Patterns and Perspectives," 2014, available at physiciansfoundation .org/uploads/default/Physicians_Foundation_2012_Biennial_Survey.pdf, 8.

10. The Physicians Foundation, "2016 Survey of America's Physicians: Practice Patterns and Perspectives," 2016, available at physiciansfoundation .org/uploads/default/Biennial_Physician_Survey_2016.pdf.

11. Kashner, Sam, "When Michael Crichton Reigned over Pop Culture, from *ER* to *Jurassic Park*," *Vanity Fair*, 2017, available at vanityfair.com

/hollywood/2017/02/michael-crichton-reign-over-pop-culture-jurassic-park
-westworld.

12. Peabody, Francis, "The Care of the Patient," *JAMA*, 88, no. 12 (1927):
877–882.

13. Jacobs, Alice K., "Rebuilding an Enduring Trust in Medicine: A Global
Mandate," *Circulation* 111 (2005): 3494–3498, available at citeseerx.ist.psu.edu
/viewdoc/download;jsessionid=3A07809804B92281B0C5B7DF27617DAC?doi
=10.1.1.493.94&rep=rep1&type=pdf.

14. Lown, Beth A., Julie Rosen, and John Marttila, "An Agenda for
Improving Compassionate Care: A Survey Shows About Half of Patients Say
Such Care is Missing," *Health Affairs* 30, no. 9 (2011): 1772–1778, available at
content.healthaffairs.org/content/30/9/1772.full.pdf.

15. Blendon, Robert J., John M. Benson, and Joachim O. Hero, "Public Trust
in Physicians—U.S. Medicine in International Perspective," *The New England
Journal of Medicine*, October 23, 2014, available at nejm.org/doi/full/10.1056
/NEJMp1407373#t=article.

16. The Physicians Foundation, "2016 Survey of America's Physicians:
Practice Patterns and Perspectives," 2016, available at physiciansfoundation
.org/uploads/default/Biennial_Physician_Survey_2016.pdf.

17. Topol, Eric, "A Doctor With A Bad Knee Runs into One-Size-Fits-
All Medicine," *The Washington Post*, December 4, 2016, available at
washingtonpost.com/national/health-science/a-doctor-with-a-bad-knee-runs
-into-one-size-fits-all-medicine/2016/12/02/d5ba55c0-a6a2-11e6-ba59
-a7d93165c6d4_story.html?utm_term=.ddb241efe94e.

18. Crichton, Michael, *Five Patients* (New York: Ballantine, 1989), 149.

19. Boër, Claudio Roberto, and Sergio Dulio, *Mass Customization and
Footwear: Myth, Salvation or Reality?* London: Springer-Verlag, 2007.

20. The Physicians Foundation, "2016 Survey of America's Physicians:
Practice Patterns and Perspectives," 2016, available at physiciansfoundation
.org/uploads/default/Biennial_Physician_Survey_2016.pdf.

21. Fonarow, G.C., E.E. Smith, J.L. Saver, et al, "Improving Door-to-Needle
Time in Acute Ischemic Stroke: The Design and Rationale for the American
Heart Association/American Stroke Association's Target: Stroke Initiative,"
Stroke, September 26, 2011.

22. Ford, Earl S., Umed A. Ajani, Janet B. Croft, Julia A. Critchley, Darwin R.
Labarthe, Thomas E. Kottke, Wayne H. Giles, and Simon Capwell, "Explaining
the Decrease in U.S. Deaths from Coronary Disease, 1980–2000," *The New
England Journal of Medicine*, June 7, 2007, available at nejm.org/doi/full
/10.1056/NEJMsa053935#t=article.

23. Donnell, Robert, "Where Has Evidence Based Medicine Taken Us in 20
Years?" KevinMD.com, June 2, 2013, kevinmd.com/blog/2013/06/evidence
-based-medicine-20-years.html.

24. Hayes, Chad, "A Taste of My Own Evidence-Based Medicine,"

ChadHayesMD.com, November 5, 2015, chadhayesmd.com/a-taste-of-my-own
-medicine.

25. Centor, Robert, "Evidence-Based Medicine: We Need to Question
Authority," KevinMD.com, November 5, 2014, kevinmd.com/blog/2014/11
/evidence-based-medicine-need-question-authority.html.

26. Brown, David, "The Keys of Nutrition," *The Washington Post*, October
22, 2002.

27. Begley, Sharon, "Records Found in Dusty Basement Undermine Decades
of Dietary Advice," STAT, April 12, 2017, available at statnews.com/2016/04/12
/unearthed-data-challenge-dietary-advice/.

28. Ramsden, Christopher E. et al., "Re-evaluation of the Traditional
Diet-Heart Hypothosis: Analysis of Recovered Data from Minnesota Coronary
Experiment (1968–73), *BMJ* 353, i1246 (2016), available at bmj.com/content
/353/bmj.i1246.

29. Gabel, J., "Ten Ways HMOs Have Changed During the 1990s," *Health
Affairs* 16, no. 3 (1997): 134–145.

30. Malone, Patrick, *The Life You Save* (Boston: Da Capo Lifelong Books,
2009), 30–34.

31. Singh, Hardeep, Ashley Meyer, and Eric Thomas, "The Frequency
of Diagnostic Errors in Outpatient Care: Estimations from Three Large
Observational Studies Involving US Adult Populations," *BMJ Quality & Safety*,
April 17, 2014 (online).

32. Verghese, Abraham et al., "Inadequacies of Physical Examination
as a Cause of Medical Errors and Adverse Events: A Collection of Vignettes,"
American Journal of Medicine 128, no. 12 (December 2015): 1322–1324.

33. Levinson, Wendy, Debra L. Roter, John P. Mullooly, et al., "Physician-
Patient Communication: The Relationship with Malpractice Claims Among
Primary Care Physicians and Surgeons," *JAMA* 277, no. 7 (1997): 553–559,
available at jamanetwork.com/journals/jama/article-abstract/414233.

34. The Physicians Foundation, "2016 Survey of America's Physicians:
Practice Patterns and Perspectives," 2016, available at physiciansfoundation
.org/uploads/default/Biennial_Physician_Survey_2016.pdf.

35. Semigran, H., J. Linder, C. Gidengil, A. Mehrotra, "Evaluation of
Symptom Checkers for Self Diagnosis and Triage: Audit Study," *The BMJ* 351,
July 8, 2015.

36. Luger, T., T. Houston, and J. Suls, "Older Adult Experience of Online
Diagnosis: Results from a Scenario-Based Think-Aloud Protocol," *Journal of
Medical Internet Research* (online), January 16, 2014.

37. American Medical Association, "AMA CEO Outlines Digital Challenges,
Opportunities Facing Medicine," AMA News Release, June 11, 2016, available at
ama-assn.org/ama-ceo-outlines-digital-challenges-opportunities-facing-medicine.

38. "No Evidence That Fitness Trackers Make You Healthier, Study Says,"
The Telegraph, February 4, 2016, available at telegraph.co.uk/technology
/2016/02/04/no-evidence-that-fitness-trackers-make-you-healthier-study-says/.

39. Topol, Eric, *The Patient Will See You Now* (New York: Basic Books), 6–7.

40. Not her real name, but instead, the pseudonym given to her by PR Web.

41. "Hurricane Sandy and Hepatitis C Won't Keep This Patient Down," BioPlus press release, November 28, 2012, available at prweb.com/printer /10171253.htm.

42. Thean, Patrick, *Rhythm: How to Achieve Breakthrough Execution and Accelerate Growth* (Austin: Greenleaf Book Group, 2014), 34.

43. "Hurricane Sandy and Hepatitis C Won't Keep This Patient Down," BioPlus press release, November 28, 2012, available at prweb.com/printer /10171253.htm.

44. Thean, Patrick et al., *Predictable Results* (Austin: Leadline, Inc., 2017).

45. Pollack, Andrew, "Hepatitis C, A Silent Killer, Meets Its Match," *The New York Times*, November 4, 2013, available at nytimes.com/2013/11/05/health /hepatitis-c-a-silent-killer-meets-its-match.html?pagewanted=all&_r=0.

46. Kliff, Sarah, "This Drug Costs $84,000 and There's Nothing the US Health-Care System Can Do to Stop It," Vox.com, December 2, 2014, vox .com/2014/12/2/7282833/sovaldi-cost.

47. Gounder, Celine, "A Better Treatment for Hepatitis C," *The New Yorker*, December 9, 2013, available at newyorker.com/tech/elements/a-better -treatment-for-hepatitis-c.

48. Cutler, David M. et al., "The Value of Antihypertensive Drugs: A Perspective on Medical Innovation," *Health Affairs* 26, no. 1 (2007): 97–110 (10.1377/hlthaff.26.1.97).

49. According to a 1976 report from the General Accounting Office, "History of the Rising Costs of the Medicare and Medicaid Programs and Attempts to Control These Costs: 1966–1975," combined spending on Medicare parts A and B and Medicaid rose from $6,381 million in fiscal year 1967 to $13,569 million in fiscal year 1971. Available at gao.gov/assets/120/112784.pdf.

50. Ibid.

51. Himmelstein, D., E. Warren, D. Thorne, and S. Woolhandler, "MarketWatch: Illness and Injury as Contributors to Bankruptcy," *Health Affairs*, February 2005.

52. Warren, Elizabeth, "Sick and Broke," *The Washington Post*, February 9, 2005, available at washingtonpost.com/wp-dyn/articles/A9447-2005Feb8.html.

53. "What Bugs Americans Most About Their Doctors," *Consumer Reports*, June 2013, available at consumerreports.org/cro/magazine/2013/06/what -bugs-you-most-about-your-doctor/index.htm.

54. The Kaiser Family Foundation and Health Research & Educational Trust, 2015 Employer Health Benefits Annual Survey, available at files.kff.org /attachment/report-2015-employer-health-benefits-survey.

55. Stanfill, Mary, Kang Lin Hsieh, Kathleen Beal, and Susan H. Fenton, "Preparing for ICD-10-CM/PCS Implementation: Impact on Productivity and Quality," Perspectives in Health Information Management, 2014, available at

perspectives.ahima.org/preparing-for-icd-10-cmpcs-implementation-impact-on
-productivity-and-quality/#.VocqEc5Op8w.

56. Williams, Mark E., "The Story of a Man Who Was a Very Good Cook,"
KevinMD.com, May 10, 2016, kevinmd.com/blog/2016/05/the-story-of-a-man
-who-was-a-very-good-cook.html.

57. Blanchfield, Bonnie B., James L. Heffernan, Bradford Osgood, Rosemary
R. Sheehan, and Gregg S. Meyer, "Saving Billions of Dollars—And Physicians'
Time—By Streamlining Billing Practices," *Health Affairs*, April 2010, available
at content.healthaffairs.org/content/29/6/1248.long.

58. The Kaiser Family Foundation and Health Research & Educational
Trust, 2015 Employer Health Benefits Annual Survey, available at files.kff.org
/attachment/report-2015-employer-health-benefits-survey; Board of Governors
of the Federal Reserve System, Report on the Economic Well-Being of U.S.
Households in 2015, May 2016, available at federalreserve.gov/2015-report
-economic-well-being-us-households-201605.pdf.

59. "Surprise Medical Bills are Costing Consumers," *Consumer Reports*,
May 8, 2015, available at consumerreports.org/cro/news/2015/05/surprise
-medical-bills-are-costing-consumers/index.htm.

60. Hamel, Liz, Mira Norton, Karen Pollitz, Larry Levitt, Gary Claxton, and
Mollyann Brodie, "The Burden of Medical Debt: Results from the Kaiser Family
Foundation/New York Times Medical Bills Survey," KFF.org, January 5, 2016,
kff.org/report-section/the-burden-of-medical-debt-section-1-who-has-medical
-bill-problems-and-what-are-the-contributing-factors/.

61. McElwee, Sean, "Enough to Make You Sick: The Burden of Medical
Debt," Demos, 2016, available at demos.org/sites/default/files/publications
/Medical%20Debt.pdf.

62. "On the Road with Steve Hartman," CBS News, August 2, 2013.

63. Renaldi, Richard, *Touching Strangers* (New York: Aperture Book
Program, Aperture Foundation, 2014), 112–114.

64. Field, Tiffany, Miguel Diego, and Maria Hernandex-Reif, "Preterm Infant
Massage Therapy Research: A Review," PMC, April 1, 2011, ncbi.nlm.nih.gov
/pmc/articles/PMC2844909/.

65. Jourard, Sidney M., "An Exploratory Study of Body-Accessibility,"
British Journal of Clinical Psychology, September 1966, available at
onlinelibrary.wiley.com/doi/10.1111/j.2044-8260.1966.tb00978.x/abstract.

66. Ofri, Danielle, "The Doctor Will See Your Electronic Medical Record
Now," Slate, August 5, 2013, slate.com/blogs/future_tense/2013/08/05/study
_reveals_doctors_are_spending_even_less_time_with_patients.html.

67. Coleman, Reid, "The Woes of Clinical Documentation: 40 Books a
Year and Counting," Nuance, February 17, 2016, whatsnext.nuance.com
/healthcare/physicians-overwhelmed-by-clinical-documentation-need-better
-technology/.

68. The White House, "Transforming Health Care: The President's Health

REFERENCES

Information Technology Plan," 2004, georgewbush-whitehouse.archives.gov /infocus/technology/economic_policy200404/chap3.html.

69. CMS, "February 2017 EHR Incentive Report," cms.gov/regulations -and-guidance/legislation/ehrincentiveprograms/downloads/february2017 _summaryreport.pdf.

70. Charles, Dustin, Meghan Gabriel, and Talisha Searcy, "Adoption of Electronic Health Record Systems Among U.S. Non-Federal Acute Care Hospitals: 2008–2014," ONC Data Brief no. 23, April 2015, healthit.gov/sites /default/files/data-brief/2014HospitalAdoptionDataBrief.pdf.

71. Gur-Arie, Margalit, "The EHR User Interface and My Personal Moment of Zen," KevinMD.com, December 2, 2012, kevinmd.com/blog/2012/12 /ehr-user-interface-personal-moment-zen.html.

72. Hill, Robert G. Jr., Lynn Marie Sears, and Scott W. Melanson, "4000 Clicks: A Productivity Analysis of Electronic Medical Records in a Community Hospital ED," *The American Journal of Emergency Medicine* 31, no. 11 (November 2013): 1591–1594, available at ajemjournal.com/article/S0735 -6757(13)00405-1/abstract.

73. Verghese, Abraham, "I Carry Your Heart," *JAMA Cardiology*, May 2016, available at http://jamanetwork.com/journals/jamacardiology/fullarticle /2515770.

74. Coan, James, Hillary Schaefer, and Richard Davidson, "Lending a Hand: Social Regulation of the Neural Response to Threat," *Psychological Science* 17, no. 12, December 1, 2006.

75. Chillot, Rick, "The Power of Touch," *Psychology Today*, March 11, 2013, psychologytoday.com/articles/201303/the-power-touch.

76. Montague, Enid et al, "Nonverbal Interpersonal Interactions in Clinical Encounters and Patient Perceptions of Empathy," *Journal of Participatory Medicine* 5, August 14, 2013.

77. Sinsky, Christine et al., "Allocation of Physician Time in Ambulatory Practice: A Time and Motion Study in 4 Specialties," *Annals of Internal Medicine*, December 6, 2016, annals.org/article.aspx?articleid=2546704.

78. Dyche, Lawrence, and Deborah Swiderski, "The Effect of Physician Solicitation Approaches on Ability to Identify Patient Concerns," *Journal of General Internal Medicine*. 20, no. 3 (March 2005): 267–270, doi: 10.1111/j.1525-1497.2005.40266.x, PMCID: PMC1490080.

79. Cohen, Susan, "The Human Whisperer," *Stanford Alumni*, January /February 2009, alumni.stanford.edu/get/page/magazine/article/?article _id=30545.

80. Chi, Jeffrey, and Abraham Verghese, "Clinical Education and the Electronic Health Record: The Flipped Patient," *Journal of the American Medical Association* 312, no. 22 (December 10, 2014): 2331–2332.

81. Kane, Leslie, and Neil Chesanow, Medscape EHR Report 2014, Medscape, Slide 19, July 15, 2014, medscape.com/features/slideshow/public/ehr2014#19.

82. Peckham, Carol, "Medscape EHR Report 2016: Physicians Rate

Top EHRs," Medscape, Slide 19, August 25, 2016, medscape.com/features /slideshow/public/ehr2016#page=19.

83. Renaldi, Richard, *Touching Strangers* (New York: Aperture Book Program, The Aperture Foundation, 2014), 9.

84. "Drama Mama," *Untold Stories of the ER*, directed by David Massar and Paul Ziller, season 9, episode 7, 2014.

85. LaMotte, Sandee, "Tapeworms and Four Other Disgusting Parasites You Should Know," CNN.com, November 8, 2015, cnn.com/2015/11/06/health /tapeworm-parasites-what-to-know/.

86. Wachter, Robert M., "How Measurement Fails Doctors and Teachers," *The New York Times*, January 16, 2016, nytimes.com/2016/01/17/opinion /sunday/how-measurement-fails-doctors-and-teachers.html?_r=2.

87. Eugenios, Jillian, "Leaving Food Uneaten May Cost You at Some Restaurants," TODAY.com, May 17, 2012, today.com/food/leaving-food-uneaten -may-cost-you-some-restaurants-778509.

88. Rice, Sabriya, "Quality Reporting's Toll on Physician Practices in Time and Money," *Modern Healthcare*, March 7, 2016.

89. Balogh, Erin, Bryan Miller, and John Ball, editors, "Improving Diagnosis in Health Care: Quality Chasm Series," report published by The National Academies of Science, Engineering, and Medicine, with contributions from the Institute of Medicine, Board on Health Care Services, and Committee on Diagnostic Error in Health Care, 2015.

90. Rice, Sabriya, "Quality Reporting's Toll on Physician Practices in Time and Money," *Modern Healthcare*, March 7, 2016.

91. Bernard, Rebekah, "A Physician's Open Letter to Medicare Patients," KevinMD.com, November 1, 2015, available at kevinmd.com/blog/2015/11/a -physicians-open-letter-to-medicare-patients.html.

92. For those not up with texting lingo, they make me shake my head while laughing my ass off.

93. Centers for Medicare & Medicaid Services, Department of Health and Human Services, Medicare Program; Merit-Based Incentive Payment System (MIPS) and Alternative Payment Model (APM) Incentive under the Physician Fee Schedule, and Criteria for Physician-Focused Payment Models; CMS-5517-P; Table 64: MIPS Proposed Rule Estimated Impact on Total Allowed Charges by Practice Size, 676.

94. Lepper, Mark, David Greene, and Richard Nisbett, "Undermining Children's Intrinsic Interest with Extrinsic Reward: A Test of the 'Overjustification' Hypothesis," *Journal of Personality and Social Psychology* 28, no. 1 (1973): 129–137, psycnet.apa.org/journals/psp/28/1/129/.

95. Soumerai, Stephen, and Ross Koppel, "Paying Doctors Bonuses for Better Health Outcomes Makes Sense in Theory. But It Doesn't Work." Vox.com, January 25, 2017, vox.com/the-big-idea/2017/1/25/14375776/pay-for -performance-doctors-bonuses.

96. Kohn, Alfie, *Punished by Rewards* (Boston: Mariner Books, 1999), 55–56.

97. Kohn, Alfie, "Why Incentive Plans Cannot Work," *Harvard Business Review*, September–October 1993, available at hbr.org/1993/09/why-incentive -plans-cannot-work.

98. As of this writing, the language quoted is now being used to promote the newest Lemony Snicket book, *File Under: 13 Suspicious Incidents*, a related book to the All the Wrong Questions series.

99. Vlaskovits, Patrick, "Henry Ford, Innovation, and That 'Faster Horse' Quote," *Harvard Business Review*, August 29, 2011, available at hbr.org/2011/08/henry-ford-never-said-the-fast.

100. Byrne, John, "A Visionary and His Limits," *Fast Company*, January 1, 2004, available at fastcompany.com/47847/visionary-and-his-limits.

101. Companion website for the PBS television special *Triumph of the Nerds: The Rise of Accidental Empires*, TV show premiered in June 1996, television show transcript Part III, Steve Jobs speaking. (Accessed pbs.org /nerds/ on March 6, 2013).

102. Markoff, John, "Apple's Visionary Redefined Digital Age," *The New York Times*, October 5, 2011, available at nytimes.com/2011/10/06/business/steve -jobs-of-apple-dies-at-56.html.

103. Butcher, Lee, *Accidental Millionaire: The Rise and Fall of Steve Jobs at Apple Computer* (New York: Paragon House, 1987). Also quoted in Malcolm Gladwell's *Outliers: The Story of Success* (New York: Little, Brown, 2008), 66.

104. Kunkle, Fredrick, "Learning to Ride Mass Transit Equals Independence for Older People," *The Washington Post*, October 11, 2015, available at washingtonpost.com/local/trafficandcommuting/learning-to-ride-mass-transit -equals-independence-for-older-people/2015/10/11/9a61bfac-6dde-11e5-aa5b -f78a98956699_story.html.

105. Bradley, Elizabeth, and Lauren Taylor, *The American Health Care Paradox: Why Spending More Is Getting Us Less* (New York: PublicAffairs, 2013), 3.

106. Wen, Leana, and Suhavi Tucker, "What Do People Want from Their Health Care? A Qualitative Study," *Journal of Participatory Medicine* 7, June 25, 2015.

107. Kaplan, G., and A. Robeznieks, "Prospering by Standardizing Processes and Improving the Patient Experience," *Modern Healthcare* 44, no. 2 (January 11, 2014): 28–29; available at modernhealthcare.com /article/20140111/MAGAZINE/301119950.

108. "VMPS Success Stories," Virginia Mason website, available at VirginiaMason.org/vmps#Success.

109. "Managing Phone Calls in Primary Care," Case Study of Virginia Mason Institute, available at virginiamasoninstitute.org/2015/03/managing-phone -calls-in-primary-care/.

110. Trimble, Chris, *How Physicians Can Fix Health Care*, American Association for Physician Leadership, 2015, from "A Note to Readers."

111. Linderman, Matt, "The Story of Polaroid Inventor Edwin Land, One of

Steve Jobs' Biggest Heros," Signal v. Noise, November 18, 2010, signalvnoise
.com/posts/2666-the-story-of-polaroid-inventor-edwin-land-one-of-steve-jobs
-biggest-heroes.

112. McElheny, Victor K., *Insisting on the Impossible: The Life of Edwin Land*, rev. ed. (New York: Basic Books, 1999), 3.

113. Berger, Warren, *A More Beautiful Question: The Power of Inquiry to Spark Breakthrough Ideas* (New York: Bloomsbury USA, 2014), 72.

114. McElheny, Victor K., *Insisting on the Impossible: The Life of Edwin Land*, rev. ed. (New York: Basic Books, 1999), 2.

115. Linderman, Matt, "The Story of Polaroid Inventor Edwin Land, One of Steve Jobs' Biggest Heroes," Signal v. Noise, November 18, 2010, available at signalvnoise.com/posts/2666-the-story-of-polaroid-inventor-edwin-land-one-of-steve-jobs-biggest-heroes.

116. The Physicians Foundation, "A Survey of America's Physicians: Practice Patterns and Perspectives," 2012, p. 8.

117. Ofri, Danielle, "Neuron Overload and the Juggling Physician," *The Lancet*, November 27, 2010, available at thelancet.com/journals/lancet/article/PIIS0140-6736(10)62157-5/fulltext?rss=yes.

118. Bush, Jonathan, "Invest for Health," Session 1, South by Southwest Interactive Conference 2016, presentation on March 14, 2016.

119. Johnson, Robert, "The Fax Machine: Technology That Refuses to Die," *The New York Times*, March 27, 2005, available at hnytimes.com/2005/03/27/business/yourmoney/the-fax-machine-technology-that-refuses-to-die.html?_r=0.

120. Mearian, Lucas, "HIPAA Rules, Outdated Tech Cost U.S. Hospitals $8.3B a Year," *Computerworld*, May 7, 2013, available at computerworld.com/article/2496995/healthcare-it/hipaa-rules—outdated-tech-cost-u-s—hospitals—8-3b-a-year.html.

121. Charatan, Fred, "US Doctors Call for Simpler Medicare Rules," *The BMJ*, March 17, 2001, 322(7287): 638, available at ncbi.nlm.nih.gov/pmc/articles/PMC1119841/.

122. Rosenbaum, Lisa, "When Doctors Tell Patients What They Don't Want to Hear," *The New Yorker*, July 23, 2013, available at newyorker.com/tech/elements/when-doctors-tell-patients-what-they-dont-want-to-hear.

123. Weeks, Jane C., et al., "Patients' Expectations about Effects of Chemotherapy for Advanced Cancer," *The New England Journal of Medicine*, 367 (2012): 1616–1625, available at nejm.org/doi/full/10.1056/NEJMoa1204410.

124. Robbins, Alexandra, "The Problem with Satisfied Patients," *The Atlantic*, April 17, 2015, available at theatlantic.com/amp/article/390684/?client=safari.

125. Sonnenberg, William, "Patient Satisfaction Is Overrated," Medscape, March 6, 2014, available at medscape.com/viewarticle/821288.

126. McCreary, Lew, "Kaiser Permanente's Innovation on The Front Lines," *Harvard Business Review*, September 2010.

127. Berger, Warren, *A More Beautiful Question: The Power of Inquiry to Spark Breakthrough Ideas* (New York, Bloomsbury Publishing PLC, 2014), 73–74.

128. "Asclepius, the God of Medicine," greeka.com, available at greeka.com /greece-myths/asclepius.htm.

129. Friedlander, Walter J., *The Golden Wand of Medicine* (New York: Greenwood Press, 1992), chapters 7 and 8.

130. Ibid., p. 153.

131. Shetty, Anil, Shraddha Shetty, and Oliver Dsouza, "Medical Symbols in Practice: Myths vs Reality," *Journal of Clinical Diagnosis and Research for Doctors* 8, no. 8 (August 2014): PC12–PC14, doi: 10.7860 /JCDR/2014/10029.4730, PMCID: PMC4190767.

INDEX

ABOUT THE AUTHOR

Halee Fischer-Wright is a nationally recognized health-care executive, physician leader, and former business consultant whose work focuses on innovation and creating cultures of excellence. Dr. Fischer-Wright is president and CEO of Medical Group Management Association (MGMA) and is the coauthor of *Tribal Leadership*, a *New York Times* best seller.

Prior to assuming her current role, she was a practicing physician, management consultant in multiple industries, president of Rose Medical Group, and chief medical officer within Centura Health. She is the recipient of multiple national awards for leadership in innovation, health care, business, and women's leadership.

Dr. Fischer-Wright holds a bachelor's degree from the University of Colorado, a master's degree in medical management from the University of Southern California, and a certificate in executive leadership coaching from Georgetown University. She received her MD from the University of Colorado. She currently lives in Denver, Colorado, with her physician husband and her two amazingly spoiled dogs.

DrHalee.com | @DrHalee
MGMA.com | @mgma

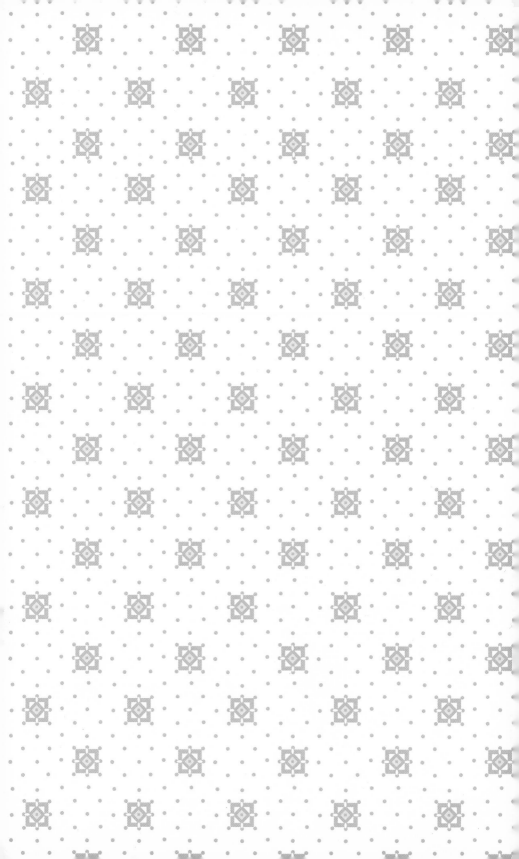